Love, Laugh, and Eat

LOVE LAUGH and EAT

And Other Secrets of Longevity from the Healthiest People on Earth

JOHN TICKELL, M.D.

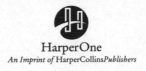

HarperOne
An Imprint of HarperCollinsPublishers

HarperOne

This book is written as a source of information only. The information contained in this book should by no means be considered a substitute for the advice of your qualified medical professional, who should always be consulted before beginning any new diet, exercise, or other health program.

LOVE, LAUGH, AND EAT: *And Other Secrets of Longevity from the Healthiest People on Earth.* Copyright © 2013 by Dr. John Tickell and Longevity Plus Pty Ltd. All rights reserved. Printed in the United States of America. No part of this book may be used or reproduced in any manner whatsoever without written permission except in the case of brief quotations embodied in critical articles and reviews. For information address HarperCollins Publishers, 10 East 53rd Street, New York, NY 10022.

HarperCollins books may be purchased for educational, business, or sales promotional use. For information please e-mail the Special Markets Department at SPsales@harpercollins.com.

HarperCollins website: http://www.harpercollins.com

HarperCollins®, 📖®, and HarperOne™ are trademarks of HarperCollins Publishers.

FIRST EDITION

Designed by Terry McGrath
Photographs courtesy of the author

Library of Congress Cataloging-in-Publication Data
Tickell, John.
Love, laugh, and eat : and other secrets of longevity from the
healthiest people on earth / John Tickell. — First edition.
    pages cm
Includes index.
ISBN 978–0–06–228622–2 1. Health behavior. 2. Longevity.
3. Nutrition. 4. Beauty, Personal. I. Title.
RA776.9.T528 2013
613.2—dc23   2013016245

13 14 15 16 17 RRD(H) 10 9 8 7 6 5 4 3 2 1

Thank you to my inspiration—
the longest-living, healthiest people on earth

Thank you to Sue, the best wife,
the best mother, and my best friend in the world

Contents

Introduction

The world is full of specialists, technical experts, and people who love to complicate things. There is a minefield of misinformation out there that confuses us about how to cope with life. Exercising, eating, and getting our brains in gear have somehow become mysteries. Well, if I have any ability as a doctor, it is the ability to simplify complicated things.

Patients generally fall into two distinct groups: the single-cause patients and the multiple-cause patients. The former are those with an obvious medical or surgical emergency—a bacterial infection, for instance, or an injury as a result of a trauma or accident, such as a broken bone. Something that "good ol' Doc" can help. The latter group, however, consists of patients with severe lifestyle ailments and diseases, such as stress, anxiety and depression, most heart diseases, type 2 diabetes, cancer, and many other ailments. The causative and precipitating factors are multiple—in most cases, researchers mumble about genetics and so on—but perhaps the real culprits are the lousy foods most of us eat, our inactivity, the environmental pollutants (including radiation) we're subjected to, and how pressured, unhappy, and dissatisfied most of us are.

This shouldn't really come as a surprise. We're always busy, and our lives are filled with stresses and strains. On top of that, we're all up against an enormous number of people and entities that don't care about our best health interests. You know who I mean; you know who I'm talking about. Fast-food restaurants, for instance, and clever companies that sell us the latest "healthy" cookies and muffins and chips. Uninformed healthcare providers are in the mix too—and so many others.

Well, despite all this, I'm here to teach you how you can love, laugh, and eat your way to the ripe old age of 100.

You're probably saying to yourself right now, "Hey, Doctor, that's impossible." But I want you to know that it *is* possible. My research over 25 years has shown me many people in their 60s, 70s, 80s, even 90s and beyond, who are younger in body and in mind, slimmer, happier, and healthier than many 40-year-olds. Believe me, it is possible. I constantly devour scientific papers and data, and with my two medical doctor children, we have traveled and watched and learned from real people in a total of more than 100 countries around the world—all to give you the best information available. Through my travels, I've learned the tried-and-true tools and techniques of longevity from the healthiest people on earth: the Okinawans, inhabitants of a large group of islands off Japan's southernmost point.

Everyone needs heroes in their life, and my heroes are the Okinawans. The Okinawans have the greatest number of centenarians per capita in the world. Okinawans enjoy longer, healthier lives—lives mostly free of heart disease, strokes, and cancer. Only 6 in 100,000 women, for instance, die from breast cancer in Okinawa. If we look at the *incidence* of breast cancer rather than the *death rate,* more than 1 woman in 10 develops breast cancer in the United States. Okinawans are the longest-living, healthiest, happiest people on the planet. How do they do it? Why are they so lucky? Personally, I don't call it luck. I call it common sense.

A world-class team of researchers set out to find out what gave the Okinawans their health advantage. Over a 25-year period, from the mid-1970s to 2001, researchers aligned with and funded by the Japan Foundation for Aging and Health—and with help from the Mayo Clinic, Harvard University, the University of Toronto, the Medical Research Council of Canada, and the Ryukyu University Hospital in Japan—examined 600 Okinawan centenarians, and lots more young people in their 80s and 90s. That's right: *young* people in their 80s and 90s. Imagine that!

Known as the Okinawan Centenarian Study, the research found that elderly Okinawans have cleaner arteries and a lower number of hormone-dependent cancers than their younger American counterparts, and their bones are stronger. Similarly, Okinawans' brains stay younger longer. In the United States, dementia usually starts around middle age—earlier than in Okinawa—and accelerates at a more rapid pace. Note the chart on page 4 showing Okinawans' level of dementia as they age compared with ours. Look at the striking differences in the older people. Amazingly, Okinawans remain younger longer, while we get older quicker.

In addition to these findings, the study overturned a conventional belief about longevity. Contrary to what you've probably been told, longevity has less to do with heredity than most people realize. Genetics, it turns out, accounts for only about 30 percent

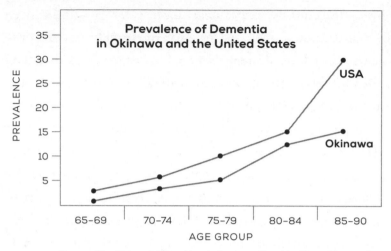

Source: *The Okinawa Way: How to Improve Your Health and Longevity Dramatically* by Bradley Wilcox, M.D., Craig Wilcox, Ph.D., and Makoto Suzuki, M.D. New York: Penguin, 2001.

of our health and life span. The overwhelming other 70 percent is the result of specific lifestyle factors such as physical activity, eating habits, and social interactions. It's these factors that explain why the Okinawans enjoy such long, happy lives. They don't care about carbs or high-protein diets or Jenny Craig. They've never counted calories or ounces or grams of fat, and they've never been lazy enough to have food delivered to their door. Nor do they take "magic pills" or drink "miracle shakes" to replace real food at meal times. They're not just built better (genetics); they also *live* better.

Now, I don't expect you to live exactly like the Okinawans. Our lives are very different from theirs. I do, however, expect you to approach their ideals and shift your brain to a New Normal. It's time to rethink the phrase "life expectancy" and change it to "health expectancy." Not how long you think you're going to *live*, but how long you expect to *be healthy*. Just like the Okinawans.

This book is designed to help you do just that. I've boiled down all the research and the principles of these wonderful people into a practical, doable everyday program to help you change your life.

All you need are the right tools and techniques. And I've already done the hard part by coming up with my ACE protocol: Activity, Coping, and Eating. The magic is in the combination of all three. Concentrating on one alone just doesn't work. You need all three to be successful; you need to involve your whole body, your mind, and what you put in your mouth. It's all tied together. Throughout the book, I show you how to incorporate each skill into your daily life.

Let's orient ourselves by looking at the drawing below. As the drawing shows, there are three parts to the human body. Arms, legs, head, mouth, nose, eyes, ears, blood vessels, organs —forget all that stuff you learned in high school anatomy and biology class. There are only *three* parts. Below the neck, that's the biggest part of the human body. That's for moving: the *A* (for Activity) part of

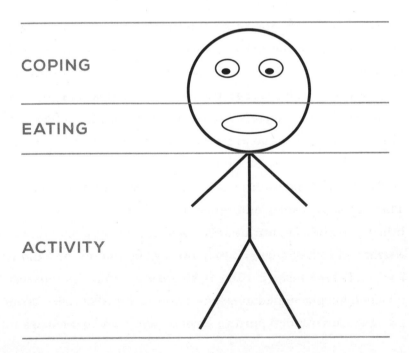

COPING

EATING

ACTIVITY

the ACE protocol. The *C* (for Coping) is the little bit from your nose up to the top of your head, which is used for thinking and stress management. And that little tiny bit in the middle is for speaking and eating, the *E* (for Eating) part of the protocol. ACE: all three parts matter.

The difference between my program and diet programs is simple: it works. I recently read a newspaper report that said 95 percent of all diets fail. Why do they fail? Because most diets deal with only one aspect—just activity (which is often "over the top" exercise) or just coping (which often adds stress rather than reducing it) or just eating (which ranges from near-starvation to miraculous, just-invented magic bullets)—but not all three at once, as my program does. We all need a coach, someone to help us along the way, someone to encourage us to succeed, help us win the game all the way to the end of the fourth quarter—which in this case means we're younger, slimmer, and filled with energy. Fad diets and other programs take you to the first or maybe second quarter. My program helps you win the whole game. The ACE program has a success rate, not a failure rate! By the way, the *worst* two words most failure programs use are *diet* and *exercise*. My ACE approach is *not* a diet—it's a wonderful, exciting *way of life* that includes good activity, good eating, and getting our brains in gear to deal with the life we would love to live.

Hundreds of thousands have already followed my techniques. They've lost tons of fat, and best of all, they're enjoying life to the fullest. Take Debby, for instance. Debby was worried about her weight and lack of energy. She was over 300 pounds and didn't feel good about herself. Then Debby decided to become part of my Love, Laugh, and Eat program, and it changed her life. As she put the ACE skills into practice, she lost weight and gained fitness

Asian and American Diets		
Intake	Asian Study	USA
Total Fat (% of calories)	14%	36–38%
Fiber (grams per day)	33	12
Total Protein (grams per day)	64	91
Animal Protein (% of total calories)	0.8%*	11%

*In this study, Asian protein is nonfish, but the bottom line is that Americans consume about 15 times more meat and dairy than Asians, and this correlates with the *frightening* incidence of artery disease, heart attacks, and strokes, as well as colon cancer, breast cancer, and prostate cancer.

Source: *The China Study: The Most Comprehensive Study of Nutrition Ever Conducted and the Startling Implications for Diet, Weight Loss, and Long-Term Health* by T. Colin Campbell and Thomas M. Campbell II. Dallas, TX: BenBella Books, 2004.

and confidence. Still on the program now, and 130 pounds lighter—remember, it's a *lifestyle* change—she gets plenty of praise from her family and her friends, and that makes her feel good and motivates her to succeed.

The ACE program is not difficult to follow. Debby learned to be active every day—that's the *A* in ACE. Her brain began thinking good things, not bad thoughts—that's the Coping, or *C,* in ACE. And she was eating delicious, health-promoting food—that's the *E* in ACE. What happened to Debby won't necessarily happen to you, but I want you to give these ACE skills a real try. Personally, I'm about to turn 70, and my passion is to celebrate life and celebrate maturity, not worry about or be afraid of getting on in years. Does that sound good to you? Yes? That's what I thought.

In my 40 years in medical practice, I've probably heard every single excuse in the book. You know, "Ah, sorry, Doc, this is just not right for me." Or "I'm too overweight to start." Or "Doc, I've tried every diet. None of them work." Or "I'm too busy—and besides, I can't afford it." I mean, I've heard *everything*. I even

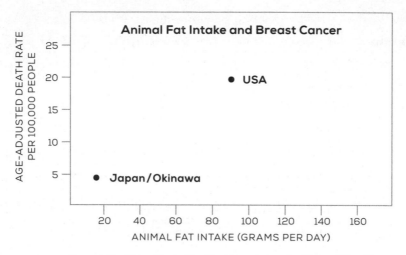

Source: *The China Study: The Most Comprehensive Study of Nutrition Ever Conducted and the Startling Implications for Diet, Weight Loss, and Long-Term Health* by T. Colin Campbell and Thomas M. Campbell II. Dallas, TX: BenBella Books, 2004.

heard this excuse once, "I don't live in Okinawa," as if it were too late or too difficult for the patient to change. Well, if you're reading this right now, it's *not* too late. It's too late only when you're lying flat in a box, and I want to make that as far away as possible from now. So no more excuses for you. I mean, you do want to lose those extra pounds, don't you? You do want to pop out of bed in the morning with the energy you had in your 20s and 30s. You do want to get through your day with less pain (or even no pain), and you want a good night's sleep, no pills—right? And wouldn't it be nice to add a little zip to your love life?

These changes are all possible if you use my ACE tools and techniques. You can do it. And the only magic is in the combination—Activity, Coping, and Eating all working together.

If you need more convincing, how about lowering your risk of prostate cancer, breast cancer, diabetes, and heart attack? Let me give you a few statistics. Today alone, at least 100 Americans died from breast cancer. Tomorrow, nearly 100 men in the United States will die from prostate cancer, 150 people from colon (or bowel) cancer. In the next hour, 100 Americans will have a heart attack. In the next *hour*. Raise your hand if you want to reduce your risk of these dreaded diseases. Yes! Now raise your hand if you want to be one of the 100 who have a heart attack in the next hour. No, I thought not. No one wants to suffer a heart attack, but we're more than willing to put terrible food into our system again and again and again, and remain inactive and not cope very well with life, which can drastically raise the likelihood of a heart attack.

This is not brain surgery. This is not rocket science. This is very attainable, practical information and tools that can become part of your normal lifestyle. I remember when an interviewer asked George Burns on his 100th birthday, "What does your doctor say about you still puffing away on a cigar now and again?" He replied, "My doctor's dead."

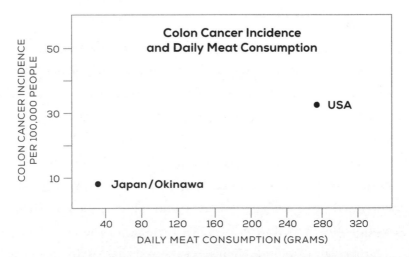

Source: *The China Study: The Most Comprehensive Study of Nutrition Ever Conducted and the Startling Implications for Diet, Weight Loss, and Long-Term Health* by T. Colin Campbell and Thomas M. Campbell II. Dallas, TX: BenBella Books, 2004.

Of course, I'm not suggesting that you should smoke cigars, but Love, Laugh, and Eat is not a fanatical approach. It's moderation, and moderation is part of the Okinawan culture—well, moderation in everything except laughter, sex, vegetables, and fish. No particular order. And never all together—it makes a heck of a mess. I promise that ACE can work for you, just as it has for the many thousands of people who have a new body and a new life because of it.

What a fabulous word, "life." *L-I-F-E: life.* What would happen, though, if we took the *F* out of *life*? Well, we'd have a *lie*, wouldn't we? There are millions of people out there living a lie because all the relevant *F*s have gone out of their *life*. So let's put some *F*s back into yours: family, fun, friendships, faith. And as the Okinawans do: fiber, fish, fruits (and vegetables). And fitness, for good measure.

Why am I so positive about the Okinawan way? Two reasons:

1. It's *not* a diet; it's a way of life.
2. It helped save my life.

I was diagnosed with inoperable brain cancer some years ago. The doctors found five tumors in my brain, all of which were malignant. One was the size of a golf ball (I'm not sure which brand!), which sounds pretty formidable. The neurosurgeons ruled out surgery because the tumors were all dangerously close to centers of critical brain function. For the next several months, I endured an intensive regimen of triple chemotherapy. When the doctors told my wife that my hair would fall out, she told them, "You can't kill barbed wire."

The specialists told me their tests showed that, apart from the cancer, my health status was good—way better than average for a person of my age. My health was probably good enough to withstand the heavy doses of triple chemo, they reasoned—which proved to be true. If I had been overweight or diabetic, they said, the chemo itself most likely would have killed me. The combination of activity, good eating, and strong mind that the ACE program had ingrained in me now gave me a fighter's chance against a formidable opponent.

A few months later, all those nasty malignant tumors were gone.

When it comes to loving life, trimming off excess pounds, and having more energy, the choice is yours. You can go the standard way with its 95 percent failure rate, or you can go the Okinawan way with its 95 percent success rate. The standard way gives us more than 100 heart attacks an hour, 30,000 breast cancer deaths each year, 5,000 new type 2 diabetics every day, and countless diagnoses of anxiety and depression.

If you agree that it is a reasonable aim to Love, Laugh, and Eat your way to 100 and have a better chance of being free from disease along the way, then we need to determine your bottom line. What do you want, and how badly do you want it?

Do you want to:

- Look better?
- Feel better?
- Sleep better?
- Love better?

Do you want to:

- Look and feel 10YY (10 years younger)?

If you answered yes to any of these questions, you're ready to get started.

PART ONE

The ACE Program

|||||||||||||||||||||||||||||||||||||||||||||||||||||||||||||||||||||||||||||||||||||||||||||||

Chapter 1

The *A* in the ACE Program—Activity

*W*e don't walk enough. We don't lift enough. We don't move enough.

The human body contains approximately 600 muscles, 180 joints, and more than 200 bones, and we make use of hardly any of them. What happens to a piece of machinery when we don't use it for long periods of time? What happens to a car if you don't turn over its engine every now and then? It starts to rust. It starts to break down. It starts to become useless. It gets old fast—even though it doesn't *wear* out. Well, our body—the greatest, most efficient machine ever invented—is no different. If you don't move your body, it rusts. It gets older faster.

Rusty people end up in rest homes, with sagging beds and uncomfortable chairs that bend their spine the wrong way. They read books and watch TV for hours on end, falling asleep in the daytime and unable to sleep at night. To get to sleep, and then to get going in the morning, they take more and more pills. Is that what we mean by "living"?

In the islands of Okinawa, there are *no* rest homes!

Inactivity creeps up on a person: the system gradually starts to shut down, then completely stops working. To prevent your body from shutting down, you have to stay active. You have to rev the engine every now and again, then put it into gear and spin the wheels.

Look in the mirror tonight. Ask yourself: Is this still the most magnificent machine on earth? I doubt that you'll say yes. And if you don't know the answer, get a second opinion.

When most people hear the word "exercise," they say, "Oh, no, it's going to be too hard." That's why I call the first element of the ACE program Activity. It's not necessarily exercise. On my program, I'd like you to eventually be climbing 200 stairs each day. People say, "Seriously—200? That's a lot of stairs." I say, "Why don't you start with 5, and then tomorrow do 10, and the next day 15, and soon you'll be climbing 200 stairs." *Activity.* Nothing fanatical, only regular activity in moderation. "But I've got arthritis," you say. Well, can you climb 2 stairs today? Hang on to the rail. Tomorrow, climb 3 stairs. "It would hurt," you counter. Then go and do some walking through water in the rehab pool down at the swimming pool. "That's too far away!"

Is it?

The end of your life is getting closer than you think!

Kenneth H. Cooper, a doctor and former colonel in the U.S. Air Force, introduced aerobics to the American public in 1968 with the publication of his groundbreaking book *Aerobics*. He stressed the importance of improving cardiovascular health through regular activity. A few years later, he established the Cooper Institute, a nonprofit center dedicated to fitness research and professional education. It was an honor and a privilege for me to meet Dr. Cooper in Dallas, Texas, at the Cooper Institute. He and the institute published an influential study on how moderate exercise, over a sustained period of time, lowered blood pressure and cholesterol and, most important, slowed down the aging process. Did you get that? Simply by staying active, you can slow down the aging process. That is amazing—and so simple.

I'll let you in on a little secret. You only have to exercise for 1 percent of your life. One-third of the ACE program demands only a minimum (dose) of 1 percent of your life. What? That *can't* be right. I mean you'd need to do more, wouldn't you? No, you don't. Think about it. There are 168 hours in a week. What's 1 percent of 168? A paltry 1.68. That's 1.68 hours, or 100 minutes. That's it. Only 100 minutes a week, or four 25-minute sessions. You can't find the time for four 25-minute sessions a week? Are you serious about that?

Think about it another way. How many hours do you sleep a night? On average, most people sleep about 7 hours out of 24, which means the average person is awake 17 hours a day—or 34 *half* hours. Over the course of a week, the average person is awake for 238 half hours. You can't find 4 or 5 or 6 of these 238 half hours a week to get moving? Again, are you serious? Do you have any respect for yourself, your partner, your children?

Do you have any idea what your peak age of physical potential is? According to Dr. Cooper, it's actually early to mid-30s, but we Americans peak in our midteens, then go backward from there. How sad is that? Once you hit 25 or 30, if you don't move a muscle every 48 hours, that muscle starts to disappear. What's worse, most of us replace 7 to 10 pounds of muscle with 7 to 10 pounds of fat every decade. *Every decade.* Similarly, once you hit 30, if you don't bang your bones on the ground every day and take them for a walk, the calcium leaves town. When calcium in

---

[Back Health]

Way back in time we humans stood up. We probably weren't meant to, as we were too busy swinging from the trees, but we *did* stand up on two legs—and in doing so we put pressure on the lower back, which means that certain activities, especially running, sometimes hurt the back.

If your body is capable of running, that's fine, but for most people starting out on an activity program, running is a bad idea. Even with walking, your back is very vulnerable, so go buy a pair of shoes with good support in the heel. Even though they may cost a fair slice of money, they'll last you for years. When you wear an excellent pair of shoes, they gently tip you forward and you're almost walking anyway. It's a great investment.

Another quick tip. Never stand around for long periods of time, because this is really bad news for the back. When you *have* to stand, do so with one foot on a step or stool—this changes the curve of the lower back a bit. And switch feet often. Or stand backward against a wall (with your feet out a couple feet in front of you) and press your lower back against the wall for a few seconds. Then, if you wish, gently roll your back slightly from side to side against the wall. This feels good.

bones is depleted, osteoporosis sets in, and your bones break more easily—wrists, hips, spinal vertebrae! A disaster, and often our own fault.

So here's what I want you to do every day. Move your 600 muscles, breathe easy, and relax often. Move your bones around a bit, and gently knock them on the ground by taking them for a walk. That stimulates calcium retention and bone regrowth.

We want you to get your heart and lungs working, get your muscles and joints moving, and get more oxygen into your brain so you can think smarter. To do that, you've got to get puffing. And there's nothing easier than walking to get lightly puffing. Walking is brilliant exercise. It's definitely a contender for the Exercise Gold Medal.

Once you've built up to the stage where you feel like you could break into a jog, try it. But jog slowly, with more of a shuffle action—no high knee action—and lean forward. With that technique you take the weight and jarring mainly through the stomach muscles rather than your back. Try walking 100 yards, then shuffle-jogging for 5 or 10 yards; then walk 100 yards again. This protects your back if you get clever at it, whereas even plain walking can put strain on the back if you're very upright. A combination of walking and gentle jogging is a good idea, as long as it's comfortable for your back. Remember, though: it's not how far you go, but the time taken to exercise.

Another good exercise is climbing stairs, which burns the equivalent of about 500 to 600 calories an hour. That's less than running but more than walking or slow jogging. It doesn't take a lot of stairs—maybe 100 or 200, depending on your pace. But speed and quantity are not the point of the exercise. The point is to tone and strengthen your quadriceps, your body's biggest muscles.

Strong quadriceps help with balance, which becomes more and more important as we get older.

So stair climbing is sensational as a preventive measure against broken bones and other major injuries of the spine. Just don't forget to use the handrail, just in case. And *do not* climb 200 stairs on Day 1. Start with 6, 7, or 8, and add 2 every day until you get to 200. How does that sound? Easy, right?

‖‖‖

TICKELL TIP

Climb 200 stairs every day. "That's a lot of stairs," you say." No, it's not. It's 10 times 20 or 20 times 10 spread out during the day. Start with 3 or 4 stairs and add 1 every half day until you're up to 50 each half day. If you're struggling, take it easy. If you're lightly puffing, that's okay. If you experience chest or neck pain, *stop immediately.*

‖‖‖

Aerobics in the gym can be a problem, especially if you're not used to much activity. Start off slowly; then, after a few sessions, begin to build up to about 20 to 30 minutes of mild- to moderate-intensity workout. The people who do up to an hour of intense pounding—pounding their back and their shins into dust—usually experience a lot of injuries.

If you're not into walking or running or stair climbing, riding a bike and swimming are also fantastic. They take the weight off the joints, get your heart ticking, and get (then keep) you toned.

There is a slight downside with swimming, however. The more efficient you become at swimming, the fewer calories you burn. This means that you need to go farther or faster to have the same calorie-burning effect. I can prove this. Go down to the local pool and watch the swimmers. If there are any large men in the group, notice how they glide through the water, lap after lap. Despite their strong motions, they aren't burning many calories. Large mass, large motion. That's why boats float. It's Archimedes's principle!

From an activity perspective, it's better to be a "bad" swimmer, because you burn more calories.

Before you undertake any new activity program, you should assess your current fitness. If you want to improve your body's internal engine, you need to get some baseline data. You have to know where you're coming from to measure how you're improving and where you're going to end up. This is true in every facet of life—whether it's a business system, an office system, a computer system, or a cardiovascular system in need of improvement.

One of the best ways to collect data about a person's fitness is to get him or her on a treadmill, strap on a pulse rate monitor, a cardiograph machine, and an oxygen consumption monitor, and then turn on the treadmill. This common assessment, known as the treadmill test, accumulates valuable baseline data about a person's pulse rate and cardiac fitness.

If you're out of shape, the treadmill test is relatively speedy because your heart rate rises quickly. After you walk for only about four minutes, you'll probably reach your maximum pulse rate. If you're a slob with a resting pulse rate of 80 or 90, all you have to do to get lightly puffing is get out of your chair; that level of activity gives your heart such a fright that it goes straight to 130, because it was almost there to start with. Conversely, a fanatical exerciser or a marathon runner would have to run on an inclined treadmill for 10, 12, or 14 minutes, because his or her heart would be stronger and thus would take longer to get to its maximum capacity.

I once tested an obese 47-year-old man on the treadmill. A computer expert, this man was stressed to the eyeballs and smoked 40 cigarettes a day. He walked into my clinic on his way to lunch.

[Pulse Rate]

Let's talk briefly about your pulse. You know what the pulse rate is, right? It's the same as the heart rate—that is, the number of times in a minute that your heart beats. To take your pulse, place two fingers at the wrist or at one side of the neck or temple. Leave your fingers there, feeling the pulse beats, and then count for 10 seconds. Multiply the number you get by 6. This is your pulse rate per minute.

(Why the fancy math—why not just count for a minute? If you're exercising and you stop and take your pulse for a whole minute, you'll get a falsely low reading, because your pulse will slow down as you're counting. Counting for a shorter time and multiplying as described above is more accurate.)

Your *maximum* pulse rate is the fastest your heart can beat. If you're on a racquetball court or squash court, for instance, and you're really going for it, sweating like hell, your maximum pulse rate is probably about 220 minus your age. So if you're 40 years of age, your pulse rate at maximum exertion is most likely 180, or 220 minus 40. A pulse rate of zero means you're dead.

Your *resting* pulse rate will be considerably lower. Perhaps the best time to take that rate is after you've gotten up in the morning and settled down for breakfast. Not as soon as you jump out of bed, because your pulse rate is often a little higher when you first start moving. Sit at the breakfast table, take your pulse for 10 seconds, and multiply by 6. The resting pulse rate in

His company had sent him as part of a new health-assessment program they were running for their employees. The man put on brand-new track shoes that he'd bought on the way to the test—sparkling new shoes, never before worn, their stripes still vibrant. I showed him onto the treadmill and connected him to the various

a physically fit person is generally somewhere between 55 and 75. In this case, 60 is better than 70; the lower rate means your heart is fitter.

Women typically have pulse rates a little higher than men because (1) women's hearts are smaller and (2) women carry a little more body fat than men. The difference in pulse rates between the two sexes is maybe 10 beats per minute.

A small subgroup of top athletes have a resting pulse rate in the high 20s or 30s, but I think that's too low. Someone with such a low rate has to work out too hard to get lightly puffing. A slob, on the other hand, or a heavy coffee drinker, or a chronic smoker, or all of the above, will most likely have a resting pulse rate in the 80s or 90s, nearly twice as high as a strong athlete per minute. But that presents a different problem—or 100,000 to 10 million problems, to be precise. A resting pulse rate that's 10 beats higher per minute than it needs to be if your heart is healthy means an extra 100,000 times a week that your heart muscle needs to contract! It's going to get tired. That's more than 5 million extra beats a year—or twice that (10 million) if your resting rate is 20 beats too high—which taxes the body and saps you of energy.

Intense exercise, however, *can* cause your heart to *stop* if your heart is not used to banging away that hard. So do *not* run out and play a hard game of racquetball unless you've played the game often since you were young.

machines and monitors. Standing still, before he even moved, the man had a resting pulse rate of 98—unbelievable! That's 98 beats every minute just to keep him alive!

I was concerned. I knew from my data that the minimum tread-mill test time was around four minutes, but I was careful: I walked him on the treadmill quite slowly and without any incline. In just 70 seconds, his pulse rate went to almost 200! I stopped the test.

He asked why I'd pulled the plug.

"Because," I told him, "you might drop dead."

"Excellent decision," the man replied.

He had absolutely no idea the danger he was in. His whole system was so ineffective that every time some slight physical or mental pressure was added . . . *whoosh,* his heart rate could flip into a dangerous rhythm.

The treadmill test and my related workup raised a lot of questions. Why did this guy get tired every day before lunch? Why did he go out to lunch five days a week? Why did he routinely have a bottle of wine at lunch to rev himself up and get a bit of fool's energy—trying to squeeze that little bit of energy out of those grapes for the next hour—only to drift into a half sleep? I mean, this guy was totally ineffective. His elevated heart rate meant his heart was dangerously inefficient. When your heart is beating inefficiently and too fast, it doesn't have time to fill with blood between beats, which means it's pumping less blood, not more. That's right: less, not more. You get dizzy. You can faint. Your heart can even stop.

Interestingly, this man's electrocardiograph (EKG) tracing was perfectly normal before the test. Sixty seconds in, however, he showed an abnormal cardiograph tracing—what we call tachycar-dia and S-T segment depression. *I* knew he had heart disease but

[Sudden Death]

Did you know that the first symptom or sign of trouble in approximately 30 percent of people with heart disease is sudden death? And sudden death is awfully hard to cure! Two-thirds of people get a warning; the other third do not—they just put the cue in the rack and lie down.

In the United States, more than 4,000 people have a heart attack every day. One-third of them drop dead. A colleague of mine once performed static health testing on a bunch of executives—that is, testing at rest rather than on a treadmill. Here's a story for you—an executive showed up, and the doctor tapped his chest. Normal. The doctor took the executive's blood pressure. Normal. The doctor checked the man's cholesterol reading. Again, normal. Finally, the doctor had the man lie on a bench and ran an electrocardiograph on him. Normal. The executive was "healthy" as far as the testing was concerned. Delighted, he got up, put on his clothes, started to leave the clinic, and on his way out dropped dead!

After hearing the story for the first time, I asked my colleague, "What did you do?"

"We turned him around so he looked like he was coming in," he said.

he didn't, because he had never noticed any symptoms. He could have had a heart attack leaving my office, or changing a tire on his car, or rushing to catch a bus, because he wasn't aware that his heart was in such bad condition. He didn't know. Worse yet, he probably didn't care.

By the way, my executive patient was sent directly to a cardiologist, who ordered an angiogram to assess the man's condition.

An angiogram involves injecting dye into the bloodstream. As the heart fills up with dye, a special scan takes pictures that reveal the coronary arteries—the arteries in and around the heart. You've heard people refer to a "coronary," as in "He had a coronary." That means a heart attack. Most people don't know this, but the three biggest arteries that supply your heart with blood and life—your coronary arteries—are about one-fifth the width of your little finger. Not very wide at all. A "coronary" happens when one or more of those arteries are blocked.

Believe it or not, most males over 15 already have a degree of artery blockage.

How does this blockage happen? Sludge builds up gradually in everyone in the Western world over a period of time, starting in the teenage years—sometimes even earlier, depending on lifestyle. Believe it or not, most males over 15 already have a degree of artery blockage. As life goes on, if you have less than 50 percent blockage, it may not matter too much; but if you get more than 50 percent blockage, you're starting to push your luck. If you build up that sludge to a stage where there's a 70 to 90 percent blockage and you don't know it, all you need is one clot of blood to come floating down that little old artery and stop things up. Or you could have an accumulation of sludge—cholesterol, calcification—that sticks to the artery wall. Either way, that added clogging causes a complete blockage, and the lights go out. This is an especially likely outcome if your other two main coronary arteries aren't in good shape either.

Postmortems done on young American soldiers during the Vietnam War showed signs of coronary artery disease. We used to think coronary artery disease started later in life, but the postmortems on those young soldiers proved that we're bringing on heart disease in our 20s and younger.

I would not be doing my *job* unless I emphasize (as does the American Heart Association) that following the menopausal years (or time) women have as many heart attacks as men. "Doctor, you're describing/talking about my husband!" You could be right, but I'm talking about you too.

What can you do about blockages? Well, you can have what's called coronary bypass surgery if the conditions are favorable. During that surgery, surgeons take a blood vessel from somewhere else in your body and sew it onto a coronary artery to—that's right—bypass the blockage. There are other procedures as well. In some cases, a stent can be popped into the clogged artery to keep it open, and clever doctors may be able to open up an artery using laser beams.

This poor chap's angiogram showed that his right coronary artery was completely blocked, his middle artery was about 90 percent blocked, while the left artery was 60 percent blocked. He was living on four-tenths of one artery, a trickle through another, and one that was all but useless. With only localized blockages, he was a good candidate for a bypass operation. (If the coronary arteries are stuffed up all the way along, then there's nothing to bypass.) So he had the operation, started eating decent food, cut back on the booze, got a dog and walked around the neighborhood most days, lost a lot of excess baggage, changed his job, reintroduced himself to his family, and learned his kids' names all over again. Now this man is really living again.

If he could do it, then you can too—preferably *before* bypass surgery or a heart attack. The Activity section of my ACE program isn't difficult. Climbing Mount Everest—now that's difficult. Moving regularly is not. Keep at it and it gets easier. And you'll start to feel better, regardless of your shape or your age.

We really should forget about how old we are, because chronological age means little. It's physiological or "how old are you really?" age that should be the measuring stick. The human body is an amazing thing: 70-year-olds can do the same thing as 40-year-olds if they do it often enough. This is called the training effect. I've seen people dramatically reverse the ticking clock of aging *after* a heart attack simply because there is now a powerful incentive to do so. They move, they eat well, and they crank up the mind power—and while the chronological clock goes ahead 10 years, their physiological clock goes back 10. It's great stuff.

A woman in her 80s riddled with arthritis once complained to me that her doctor didn't even tell her to "exercise" until she turned 80. The water exercises she started doing at the pool freed up her joints, allowing her to move more freely, and more comfortably, than she had in years.

"Why didn't he tell me when I was 60?" she asked.

It's never too late—or too early—to get active.

II

The C in the ACE Program—Coping

When I was younger, I was fortunate to meet Hans Selye, a world-famous endocrinologist who researched how organisms respond to changes in environmental conditions and stimuli. During our conversation, he told me that most people don't really understand stress. He explained that stress is an internal phenomenon; it's how you and I and everyone else respond to outward pressure. And, believe me, there's a difference. Pressure is on the outside. Stress is on the inside; it's your *response* to a particular pressure. Pressure is universal. Your stress response is personal—it's your choice.

Pressure is universal. Your stress response is personal— it's your choice.

If you put the same pressure on six people, you'll most likely get six different responses. Same pressure, varied responses. The individual always gets to choose how he or she is going to respond. A person who generally feels good about life may respond to a particular pressure by saying, "No problem. I'm going to respond well to this. I'm going to get through it." For this person, pressure presents itself as a challenge that stimulates positive action. We should all be so lucky.

The next person, however, might crumble in the same situation. Person 1 thrives, but person 2 falls apart. Why? Because it's all in his or her heart and mind. It's an attitude and it's a feeling.

I'll say it again. Stress is internal. It's your choice what to do with the pressure—will your stress response be positive or negative?

Pressure is incredible stuff. It's both frightening and exciting. In short bursts, it's stimulating and can be productive. In long, drawn-out doses, it can be soul-destroying. When times are good, we put ourselves under tremendous pressure to succeed. When times are lousy, we put ourselves under tremendous pressure not to screw up. Life's full of pressures, good and bad. While we can't control the pressure, we can control our stress response. It's all about how we deal with it, how to use it for our benefit, and, most important, how to learn to love it.

That's why champions are champions: they perform well under pressure. Jack Nicklaus, the greatest golfer of all time, once told me that he always knew he would be able to handle the pressure of the final round of a major championship on a Sunday afternoon, while most of his competitors probably would not. Performance under pressure, or PUP, separates champions from everyone else.

One factor that plays an enormous part in how a person processes and responds to a pressure situation is the personality of that person.

[Caveman, Cavewoman, Cavepersons]

Stress was invented way back in the Dark Ages, the caveman and cavewoman ages.

Faced with an aggressive beast, the caveman or cavewoman became really scared, and what happened back then still happens now: the adrenal glands pumped adrenaline into the system.

Today, when you're faced with an intense challenge, a life-or-death circumstance, your physical and emotional response—known as "fight or flight"—is the same. The hair stands up on the back of your neck, your pulse rate increases, your blood rushes to the muscles (which then tense up for action), your mouth goes dry, and you have to make a very quick decision: Do you stay there and fight or do you run like hell?

Fight or flight? That's an adrenaline response, pure and simple. It's handy stuff, adrenaline, because it sets you up to perform tasks that you ordinarily couldn't or wouldn't perform. For example, women have been known to perform superhuman tasks, acting with an incredible show of strength, to save their endangered babies.

But what if the danger is less grave? Somebody screams at you in a traffic jam, say, and you scream back, your heart suddenly going bang, bang, bang. It would be fine if you could jump out and punch the other driver in the face, but you can't. Socially, and morally, it's unacceptable.

It would be all over, if you could. The adrenaline response would die down. Either the angry animal would kill you, or you

(continued . . .)

would kill it; or you would run and you'd be safe. Either way, the adrenaline surge would go away.

But what about this life we're in?

This is Stress City.

Things don't die down—things stay worked up. There's this situation and there's that situation—we get angry, we get frustrated, there are more pressures, there are clocks to watch and deadlines to make . . . the body just can't keep up.

Let's take a closer look at how the process works. We'll start with the adrenal glands, which sit on top of the kidneys. Adrenaline comes from the adrenal medulla, which is located toward the center of the little adrenal glands. But there is only so much adrenaline that can be squirted into the system.

When the acute stress response dies down, the initial adrenaline surge drops away. If the body is still under enormous pressure because it hasn't gotten rid of the problem, then something called the chronic stress response comes into play.

For this response, the adrenal cortex takes over—that's the outside piece of the little glands—pumping cortisone substances into the system. Cortisone is one of the wide range of steroid hormones that the body produces. You have probably also heard of anabolic steroids that athletes take to cheat. There are many different forms of these hormones that can increase performance and reduce the healing time from injuries. A form of cortisone can be a life-saving drug. For example, doctors may give it to patients in tablet, injection, or inhalation form when certain things go wrong with the skin or during an asthma attack. In patients who've had a kidney transplant, doctors may administer cortisone to subdue the immune system so that the new kidney is not rejected. Likewise, when a patient's body starts fighting itself, as with autoimmune diseases such as rheumatoid arthritis and some tissue and skin conditions, doctors may prescribe cortisone to stop the immune system being so aggressive.

Sure it dampens down the immune system, but a person can't take excessive doses of cortisone forever because it has side effects. You've probably felt them yourself, not as a response to medicine prescribed by a doctor, but as part of the chronic stress response. You stimulate your adrenal glands to increase natural levels of cortisone day after day, especially if you're lousy at coping with problems.

What are the side effects of cortisone?

You retain fluid, becoming bloated and putting on weight; your skin degenerates because its support system is wrecked, so you get little lines; your bones start to get soft; back pain sets in; you may suffer from ulcers in your mouth and even in your stomach.

It's the chronic stress response. And we do it to ourselves!

Let's say a group of runners is lined up for the final of the 100-meter sprint at the Olympic Games. The starter raises his gun, and each runner tenses on the starting blocks, all pumped up, ready to go. Suddenly the organizers decide to postpone the final until the next day because the wind is too strong.

(continued . . .)

Now, these finely tuned athletes are nervous. They've been building up to this for months or years. They're pumped up. The adrenaline is flowing in an acute stress response. They're ready to fire—then they're sent home.

What do they do? They sit around and stew.

The race organizers cancel the final the next day too, because of a bomb threat, and the day after that because of impending storms.

Talk about chronic stress!

The body can't switch off.

As the cortisone levels rise, those hormones begin to chip away at the body.

Think about it: Why do doctors give you cortisone? To dampen down the immune system.

What is your own cortisone doing to you? Destroying the immune system. Your resistance starts to fall away, and you're open to more colds, more influenza, more ulcers, more this, more that—even, dare I say it, more cancers.

When you don't cope well for long periods, allowing stress to build up, you get less healthy and illness strikes. There are just too many of these hormones racing around your body.

That's when people start going off the rails.

They say, "Yeah, well, I need more coffee, more fast foods, more cigarettes to keep me going."

Actually, they don't say it; they just do it. Eat more. Drink more. Smoke more.

Until something snaps.

You've heard of the type A personality? Type A people are generally considered ambitious. They're stubborn and may become hostile. They're fast-moving creatures. They often get aggressive when things slow down—they tap their pen on the table, their knees jiggle under the desk, and one foot goes up and down because things just aren't fast enough for them. They want everything to happen, like, *now*.

They also have a higher risk of heart attacks.

Type Bs, on the other hand, are more laid-back. Type B people feel that no problem is a *great* problem—that whatever is wrong will probably fix itself, so why bother? They're likely to sit back in their chairs in meetings, letting the type As lean forward. They're likely to be less successful, at least in the traditional, Western definition of the word. (We measure success by the numbers—how much and how many.) But type Bs are also likely to have fewer heart attacks and live longer.

I'm not really worried about type Bs. Not even so much about type As who learn how to "switch off." The type of people I worry most about are the type Cs. Type Cs often fool you because they look like they're handling the world pretty well. They tend to have a bland expression on their face. They tend to sit upright on the chair rather than forward or backward. But they're also suppressing feelings. All the pressures, fears, jealousies, problems—type Cs internalize them. They stew on them and never get things off their chest. The turmoil is all on the inside. And this has tremendous adverse effects. Did you know that science is now telling us type C people are more likely to develop cancer? I believe, and many doctors believe, that this is true.

Maybe we could all just change our attitudes a little. Maybe be more like the Okinawans, more like type B people. Type Bs are easier to please. Their level of tolerance for frustration is higher. They're calmer. As a result of all that, type B people don't have the high risk of heart attacks that type A people do. And type B people would seem less likely to develop cancer than type C people.

People argue that I can't prove this. I'm the first to agree, because, unlike cholesterol or blood pressure, it's impossible to measure and categorize behavior and responses to certain conditions over an extended period of time (although it is possible to measure levels of some stress hormones, such as blood cortisol). Nevertheless, I can type a person's behavior by talking to them for a few minutes, then observing them for a few minutes more. And, as with cholesterol or blood pressure, you can change your behavior and your reactions to pressure if you want to.

My question to you is, Why *wouldn't* you want to change how you process pressure and have a better stress response outcome?

Which brings us to the second part of my ACE program, Coping.

Coping is all about attitude. About your outlook on life—the way you react to different situations and the way you relate to people you love, like, and don't particularly care for. You always have a choice between reacting positively and reacting negatively to pressure. And, of course, there is a third option: just walk away.

Never let anyone tell you that all stress is bad, because it isn't. There is negative stress, which is the result of pressure you can't cope with. This kind of stress leads to overload, exhaustion, and burnout.

But there is also positive stress. This happens when challenges come at you when you're feeling well, coping well, and surrounding yourself with motivating thoughts and positive people. And this is where achievements stem from. It's very easy to lose perspective in times of extreme pressure, but extreme pressure can cause some people to do great things—in business, in sports, and in life. Champions, as we saw earlier, perform very well under pressure.

[**Warning Signs**]

What about those little warning signs of negative stress, those cracks that appear in your carefully presented persona, one by one? If you cope poorly (or not at all) for three or four days, one or more of the following warning signs will let you know that you're headed toward a breakdown.

Warning Sign 1: Muscle Spasms

People generally ignore this warning sign. Muscle spasms take different forms in different parts of the body—and they're known by various names: headache, migraine, a pain in the neck, etc. People sit at their desks all day, hunched up and stressed out. I tell them to relax. They say, "I am relaxed, but my neck's gone." I go around the back and tell them, "No, your neck's still there." It's just a spasm. Your neck is basically screaming at you. It's begging you to please jump out of the pressure cooker and become a type B for a few minutes. Just unwind and relax.

Muscle spasms a little lower down are felt as chest pain. People think they're having a heart attack. Usually, though, it's just a spasm of the muscles between the ribs due to stress. Your body once again is telling you something.

Heart pain, or angina—the sort of chest pain that is not a muscle spasm but may signify a heart attack—is usually not a sharp or stabbing pain, but rather a tightness or feeling of pressure, as if someone were tightening a huge rubber band around your chest or placing a heavy weight on it. It some-times feels like indigestion. The pain often radiates up to your neck and through your arms. Obviously, if you're uncer-tain about the pain, quickly get to the hospital or call an

(continued . . .)

ambulance. (A time delay often occurs when people attempt to contact their local health practitioner for advice. Time is critical—call 9-1-1! Some people are tempted to say, "But I'm sure it's nothing." Question: Would you rather feel silly or feel dead?)

Muscle spasms can also occur in your stomach, caused by acid increasing in that region. If acid pours into your stomach in large quantities in the middle of the night, you may wake up with abdominal pain. This may be transient, but it can also last for 30 minutes or up to an hour, sometimes longer. This might indicate that you're developing an ulcer—talk about a warning sign!

Another common sign, particularly in middle-aged men, is lower back pain. Most cases of back pain are simple muscle spasms and weak "core" muscle tone. A few days out of the pressure cooker, however, could work wonders.

Loose bowel movements in adults can be the result of spasms in the colon. Doctors often diagnose this as irritable bowel syndrome or irritable colon or some type of colitis. As with other spasms, a few days of rest and relaxation can help, but you *must* seek medical attention if the problem continues, or if there is associated pain or bleeding.

Warning Sign 2: The CATS Syndrome

Caffeine, alcohol, tobacco, and sugar. I abbreviate these as CATS. Have you ever wondered how much chemical stimulation you need to survive? How much caffeine? How much alcohol? How much tobacco and nicotine? How much refined and processed sugar? I guarantee you, it's too much. And I've added another S for good measure: sleep. Sleep disturbance is often the first sign of not coping well.

If every time you feel hassled you go to the office coffee machine and zap yourself with another shot of caffeine, you're stuck on the stimulant roller coaster. Your blood sugar goes up for 20 minutes and you feel better, but then you're down rapidly as soon as your blood sugar drops. You begin to get irritable. You get a bit depressed. You ache for another coffee. Or another cigarette. Another cookie. Just to get back up again. Don't do it. And if you're not sleeping well, don't drink caffeine after 2:00 P.M.

What's the alternative? Ever heard of a glass of water with a slice of lemon? That usually does the trick. Lemon juice helps to lower the glycemic index of carbohydrates and slows down the absorption of sugars. Where's the water dispenser in the office? Water goes in the same cup, it's liquid, it goes in the same hole in your face, and it tastes great. You don't need more than two or—maximum—three coffees a day. If you limit your caffeine intake to two cups a day, you'll feel better and you'll save up to $5,000 a year on coffee.

If you lined up all the legal drugs in the world, caffeine, alcohol, and nicotine would be the Big Three, and nicotine would come at the worst end. Smoking is probably the greatest expression of non-coping there is. There are bad drugs and not-so-bad drugs. Alcohol, for instance, can be closer to the not-so-bad end of the drug scale if consumed in moderation. In fact, alcohol can have positive effects on people, according to some researchers, particularly when it comes to releasing the pressure valve. A drink or two helps relax you. (Notice I didn't say a dozen or more drinks.) While alcohol is technically a depressant, the first couple of drinks release or take away

(continued . . .)

your inhibitions, which can be a good thing every now and again. The downside is that alcohol makes you more confident, which then makes you order another three or four drinks.

Alcohol also thins the blood, which can be quite positive. In addition, alcohol pumps up the production of certain chemicals—high-density lipoproteins (HDL)—in the blood. These substances scavenge cholesterol out of the arteries and take it back to the liver, which is very useful. So it's been shown that people who drink some alcohol *may* have a lower risk of heart disease. The other great thing about alcohol: if you have enough of the stuff, it can make ugly people look really beautiful. But alcohol is a *drug* that kills liver and brain cells. Be careful.

Warning Sign 3: Skin Problems

Many itches and rashes on adult skin are precipitated by not coping. You may have an underlying genetic predisposition to a skin problem, but the condition tends to flare up when you're under extreme, long-term pressure. It's a warning sign, plain and simple. Skin specialists have a lot of fun—nobody dies from an itch and there are no after-hour calls. They give out nice pills and lotions, which do good things; but if you take a holiday and unwind, there is often a similar effect when you suffer from tension-related skin conditions.

Warning Sign 4: Time Urgency

Look at all the people in the world who have too much to do and not enough time to do it—every day of the week. You could have too much to do for a few days or a week maybe, or perhaps you have an important project that takes two weeks in a row. That's fine. But unless you take your "B-time" (your out-of-the-pressure-cooker time) when those projects are over, you're time urgent *all* the time—and that's a huge warning. The immune system weakens under that sort of negative stress, and this can be heart attack territory.

Warning Sign 5: Hostility

A giant difference between type A maniacs who survive and type A maniacs who don't is the hostility streak.

People with that streak turn hostile when their house of cards comes tumbling down around them. But even little things irritate hostile type As—things like creaky desks, flies, odd noises, bright lights, air conditioners, papers, people, kids—everything and anything. A great measure of your tolerance level is how you handle noise. For example, when you walk into your home on any given day, your kids are probably making the same amount of noise they make every day, day in, day out. But your tolerance changes depending on your response to external pressure. Sometimes you can stand the kids' noise. Other times you cannot. *You've* changed. *They* haven't.

If you find that you're increasingly irritated in such circumstances, then it's time to jump out of your pressure cooker, or at least release some of the pressure.

It makes no sense to be aggressive all the time. If your aggression lasts only briefly, fine. But if you're constantly acting in a state of aggression, you'll start to crumble.

Warning Sign 6: Cynicism

What a warning. The normal person turned cynic. Cynics find it difficult to have positive thoughts when the pressure rises. They can't see the "opportunity in adversity." They don't realize that "every cloud has a silver lining." Cynics can't become champions!

Mountains can be made from molehills, and minor problems can become insurmountable; but champions do the opposite: they make molehills out of mountains—they climb mountains and go to the top! How well you cope with the different elements in your life can affect your physical and mental well-being, and vice versa.

As I've already mentioned, 95 percent of all diets fail. I believe it's because most people don't deal with the part of the body above their shoulders. Yet that's the most important part of the body. The size of our frontal lobe sets us apart from the animals: it's relatively bigger and more developed. Do you know what this means? It means we have choices in life. We get to make conscious decisions. This is a good feature, because the most effective way to cope with pressure is to increase your good habits and decrease your bad ones—by conscious choice.

Even more convenient is the fact that it takes only 21 days to build half a habit. Three weeks, that's it. It's all determined right there in the brain's frontal zone with choice. It's *your* choice. How do you begin to cope better? By taking action steps. Three specific steps of action, to be exact.

Step 1: Cut Down on the CATS

The CATS syndrome, as you will recall, involves caffeine, alcohol, tobacco, and refined and processed sugars. If you want to have a cup of coffee, that's fine. If you want to have a couple of cups a day, that's okay too. But if you want 10 or 12 cups a day, your blood sugar level is going to swing up and down all day. And you'll run a high risk of diabetes. Why would you do that to yourself?

And there are calories in coffee. Oh, not so much in the plain product: there's just 1 calorie in a cup of black coffee, green tea,

[Sugar in the Morning, Sugar in the Evening, Sugar at Suppertime]

Sugar is good. It's a stimulant. It gets you going, because your body uses it to produce energy. It's also in almost everything— from fruits off the tree to medicines to snacks to breakfast, lunch, and dinner.

Sugar comes in many different forms. Sometimes it's fruit sugar. Sometimes it's white crystalized sugar. Sometimes it's syrup. Sometimes it's high-fructose corn syrup, which is often blamed as the number one source of calories in the United States. Even processed (refined) carbohydrates, like bread and pasta and french fries and pretty much every other kind of popular food, can be a source of sugar. Once your body breaks down these carbohydrates, they turn to sugar, immediately increasing sugar levels in your blood- stream.

When you eat lots of refined, simple sugars—the kind found in candies, cookies and cakes, soft drinks, and pastries—your bloodstream absorbs them rapidly, ready to convert them into energy. The more refined the carbohydrate, the faster the calories move into the system.

A can of soft drink can contain up to 200 calories, giving you a jolt of energy. That's sort of okay every now and then, if you burn the energy up straightaway.

What happens, though, when you don't burn up the energy quickly? What does the body do with it? It stores it up for later use. And how does the body store most excess energy? As fat, of course! But once it's turned into fat it's harder to burn

(continued . . .)

off, because the body uses the available sugars and carbohydrates first and starts into the fat stores later on.

If you have three or four years' worth of energy stored up and hanging around your stomach and hips, that's not so good. How much does a building block weigh? Six pounds? Eight pounds? Ten pounds? Have you got two or three bricks hanging around your belly or your thighs or your backside? That's heavy stuff to carry around every day.

Two calories a minute is the maximum amount of energy you burn sitting on your backside. Energy in = energy out. The moral of the story: avoid simple carbohydrates, which is "fast sugar."

You hardly ever find a fat vegetarian. Most of their sugar intake is in complex carbohydrate forms such as whole grains, vegetables, and less-refined breads and pastas, all of which take longer to absorb.

Go for some simple sugars occasionally if you want, especially if you're very active. But a balance is smart, isn't it? While there's nothing grossly wrong with a little sugar now and again, it's crucial to define what we mean by moderation. Americans today consume about 150 pounds of sugar and 79 pounds of high-fructose corn syrup per person per year, or between 20 and 30 teaspoons of sugar a day. *That's* certainly not moderation!

This type of exposure can lead to severe metabolic consequences and can exacerbate addictive processes, which make it next to impossible to break the cycle of craving unhealthy foods and drinks.

or black tea. Grandma used to pour a little bit of milk into the coffee, which pushed it up to 15 calories. But no, we don't do that. Today, we have cappuccinos. They're 50 calories. Or we have lattes. They're 100 calories or more. People say, "Ah, but Doctor, I didn't have many." I say, "I saw that you had five today." That's 500 calories. A pound of fat equals 3,500 calories. So if you drink five lattes in a day, you're consuming 500 calories a day. That adds up to 3,500 extra calories per week. That's a pound of fat you've put on just by drinking coffee—in just one week. And that doesn't factor in the sugar. A teaspoon of sugar contains 17 calories. Two teaspoons in each of your five lattes adds another 170 calories. Which means you'll pack on another pound of fat every three weeks—just from the sugar.

TICKELL TIP

To fire yourself up, have a cup of coffee or cappuccino or black tea *once* a day at about 10:30 A.M. Sprinkle in a teaspoon of sugar if you must. If you want the cappuccino, add the teaspoon of sugar to the froth, but don't mix it in—drink the coffee through the froth. Having green tea with breakfast gets you going and starts you off "healthy," then at 10:30–*bang!* You're fired up until midafternoon.

While the human body loves a good kick now and again, whether it's from caffeine, sugar, or alcohol, you do have to be conscious about how many chemicals you're pumping into your body. Generously, two or three shots of caffeine a day are okay. So are one or two drinks of alcohol every now and again. Getting beyond that, though—4, 8, 10, or 12 cups a day, or 6, 10, or 13 drinks a day—is way too much. That's over the top. That's a warning sign. As I noted earlier, alcohol kills liver cells and brain cells.

Tobacco and nicotine, on the other hand, are total disasters. There's no acceptable moderation. With more than 200 deadly poisons in each cigarette, smoking is roughly the equivalent of extending a length of tube from the exhaust pipe of your car into your lungs and inhaling the carbon monoxide. It's suicide by cigarettes, plain and simple. There is an average life expectancy differential of seven to nine years between smokers and nonsmokers. *Fact*.

Did you hear me?

||||||||||||||||||||||||||||||||||||||||||||||||||||||||||||||||||||||||||||||

TICKELL TIP

The average smoker smokes 20 cigarettes a day
for 35 years. That's over 250,000 cigarettes—a quarter
of a million. In each one there are 200 lethal poisons,
40 of which are carcinogenic. It's impossible to be
intelligent and smoke at the same time. Stop smoking,
idiot! Let's repeat that—it is *impossible* to be
intelligent and smoke at the same time.

||||||||||||||||||||||||||||||||||||||||||||||||||||||||||||||||||||||||||||||

Step 2: Flip the Switch

The second step on the road to better coping skills is to flip the switch. What switch? The emotional-practical switch. Let's look at what that entails.

[Kicking Caffeine]

Coffee, soda additives, and alcohol are diuretics: they purge water from your body. That means you need to drink more water to compensate and to make sure your body functions at a high level.

While small amounts of coffee won't kill you, caffeine in large quantities leads to a higher risk of all sorts of health problems, such as adrenal fatigue, heart arrhythmia, coronary artery spasm, anxiety, disturbed sleep patterns, hormonal disruptions, and even maybe diabetes. If you want the high without the addiction, try chai, green, herbal, or fresh lemon and ginger teas. They are great alternatives to coffee and may even aid in weight loss and help increase immunity and robust health, especially green tea.

If you're not yet ready to give up your morning cup of coffee, make sure you stay properly hydrated. And if you can't give up sweeteners, try replacing sugar with stevia, a natural herbal sweetener from the sunflower family. It's much sweeter than sugar and has way fewer calories.

The brain has a practical side and an emotional side. The trick is to keep your brain switched to the practical side most of the time.

Emotional eating is the biggest problem most people face today. "Ah, yes," you might say, "but I'm terribly lonely, so I need to eat more." Or "I'm depressed," or "I'm stressed." Or, my personal favorite, "I eat for comfort." All these things are true, but they're also potentially helping to kill you. Instead of using food to fill some hole in your life, turn the switch to the practical side.

Who is in control of your life?

Love yourself and respect yourself. Food may be part of the answer but it's not *the* answer; your need for certain foods is just a blanket symptom. Turn the switch every day for a while. Before you realize it, you'll start to feel better about yourself. You'll have a higher self-image, and you'll respect yourself more. Just turn the switch.

The Practical Side	The Emotional Side
Respect	Comfort
Love	Anxiety
Family	Loneliness
Health	Frustration
Self-image	"I don't care"
	"That's just who I am"
	Reward
	Anger
	Depression
	Jealousy
	Hate
	Disgust
	Stress
	Boredom
	Excitement
	Sorrow
	Resignation

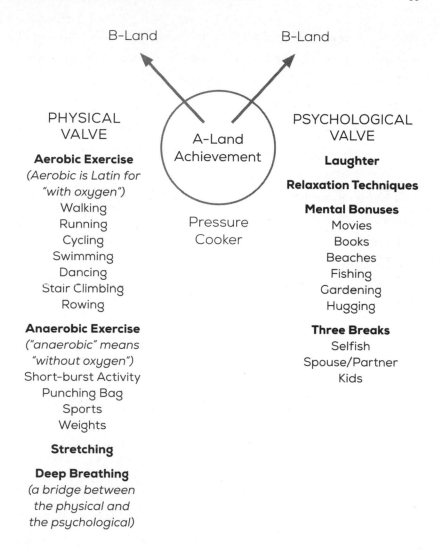

B-Land   B-Land

PHYSICAL VALVE

A-Land Achievement

PSYCHOLOGICAL VALVE

Aerobic Exercise
(Aerobic is Latin for "with oxygen")
Walking
Running
Cycling
Swimming
Dancing
Stair Climbing
Rowing

Pressure Cooker

Laughter

Relaxation Techniques

Mental Bonuses
Movies
Books
Beaches
Fishing
Gardening
Hugging

Anaerobic Exercise
("anaerobic" means "without oxygen")
Short-burst Activity
Punching Bag
Sports
Weights

Three Breaks
Selfish
Spouse/Partner
Kids

Stretching

Deep Breathing
(a bridge between the physical and the psychological)

Step 3: Escape from the Pressure Cooker

Whether we want to or not, we live in a pressure cooker. And that's fine, because a little pressure now and again is good for us. We're allowed to achieve. We're called human beens, not has-beens. And human beings love achieving. So you're allowed to put yourself under a little bit of pressure. But don't stay in the pressure cooker

8 days a week and 57 weeks a year, because eventually your world will blow up, your body will fall to bits, and your immune system will crash, leading to all sorts of health risks, including cancer, diabetes, and heart attacks.

Many of us live in A-land, where we want everything to happen immediately. Type As *love* to be in A-land. "I want it *now*." Residents of A-land run a very high risk of heart attacks. A-land is all well and good to visit every now and again, but you can't live there and remain healthy. There's just too much pressure. In fact, A-land is the ultimate pressure cooker. You need to get out of it regularly and back into B-land.

So how can you get out of the pressure cooker? There are two valves to help you release some steam, so to speak: the physical valve and the psychological valve.

The Four Aces

Life is like a game of cards: you can't be truly happy unless you hold all four aces.

The Ace of Diamonds represents the drive for wealth. If that's the only ace in your pack, you'll never find happiness. Western life is a counting game, isn't it? It's count, count, count—money, money, money. But show me people with diamonds and a heap of money, and I'll show you plenty of miserable people, whether they're multimillionaires or billionaires.

You can buy friends and you can rent friends, but unless you've got the other three aces in your pack, you're not working and playing with a full deck. You can't be truly happy without the other three.

The Ace of Hearts represents relationships, family, spirituality, belief systems, and compassion. If this is the one ace you're missing, you won't find happiness. Show me a guy with the diamonds and no heart, and I'll show you an empty person.

The Ace of Spades represents your work ethic. We all need to do some digging. We need to get our hands dirty and go the extra mile. The more you work at something, the better you get. If you're not getting better, seek help, or maybe a coach.

As we get on in years, we stop work and retire—to do what? "Retire" is a peculiar word. You're tired—why would you want to get re-tired? People who live a long, healthy, and happy life seem to keep reasonably busy. Are you involved in a charity? Are you doing good for the world?

The Ace of Clubs is the social ace. It represents social contact. People tend to forget their friends; they really do. When was the last time you hung out with your friends just for the sake of being with them, just for laughs? I bet you can't remember. You need your friends. Share a drink; tell a story. The Okinawan culture depends on support systems. Okinawans' entire way of life revolves around their connection with other people. Sociologists call it social connectedness.

If you hold the four aces in your pack, you can be truly happy. And isn't that the ultimate goal in life for ourselves and our loved ones?

It's all part of the same deal. You see, it's not the cards we're dealt in the game of life that matters. It's the way we play the game. And the best cards in the pack are those four aces.

Lots of the "pop research" that you read about in magazines suggests that our health and fate are determined by genetics. Don't you believe it! As I mentioned in the introduction, genetic influence can be suppressed as low as 30 percent. The other 70 percent is up to us. If we play our cards right, we end up with the aces.

Oh, and don't forget the jokers in your pack. See the funny side of life. Have a laugh. It's great medicine—one of the best ways to cope.

||||||||||||||||||||||||||||||||||||||||||||||||||||||||||||||||||||||||||||||||||||||||||||||||||||||||

Chapter 3

The *E* in the ACE Program—
Eating

*W*e Americans indulge in the world's worst eating habits. We eat out often. We get takeout because it's easy and cheap. It's no wonder we're fat. Our food's full of animal protein and grease, and its nutritional value is often close to zero.

The standard American diet is more than 50 percent meat and dairy, with more than half of the rest consisting of processed and refined junk. We wonder why we're getting diabetes, heart attacks, and breast cancer earlier and earlier in life.

Given our eating habits, it's no wonder we spend millions and millions of dollars every day on diet books, yet all diet books seem to say something different. One says this; another says that. While we readers get confused, the authors get wealthy. I don't know who invented the word "diet," but if we could find that person, we should banish him or her forever, because "diet" is a four-letter word.

I have to say it again: valid research tells us that diets have a 95 percent failure rate. Most people who go *on* a diet go *off* the diet again before it makes any lasting difference. The success of a diet is measured after three years—not three days or three weeks, which is the life span of most diet efforts.

Valid research tells us that diets have a 95 percent failure rate. Most people who go ON a diet go OFF the diet again before it makes any lasting difference. The success of a diet is measured after three years—not three days or three weeks, which is the life span of most diet efforts.

When you go on a diet, you want some action, some visible results. You want to lose weight as fast as you can. Unfortunately, when you lose weight fast, a lot of what you're losing is fluid. I'll tell you a secret. On some weight loss shows, contestants lose huge amounts of weight in the first week, and most of it is fluid. A pint of water weighs about a pound, so if you drink eight pints of water (in other words, a gallon) before you weigh in, you weigh eight pounds heavier. This is easy to lose in the first week, but it's *not* fat loss. Then, if you're like most dieters, as you finally begin to lose fat you lose muscle as well—and the faster the weight comes off, the more muscle bulk you lose. Then, tired of depriving yourself, you put weight back on within a few weeks or months. You put back on the fluid and the fat. The only thing you *don't* put back on is all of the muscle that has disappeared. You're back at square one, but your percentage of body fat is actually higher than when you started!

One thing I've noticed is that the more time people spend thinking about food, talking about food, reading about food, and preparing food, the heavier or more frightfully thin these people are. They're too far on one end of the spectrum, either way.

We make things harder for ourselves, simply because of how we eat. Food doesn't have to be this complicated. In fact, food is *simple*.

He or she is a "good cook." What does that even mean? It means fancy pans and lots of additives, like butter, cream, sauces, and gravies. In my mind, it also means a cook who is likely to be overweight. Lots of celebrity chefs are overweight. Ever wonder why? Mixing, stirring, tasting, more cream, more fat, more this, more that.

A really good cook is a healthy cook.

It's impossible to sustain healthful eating until you realize one important fact: a meal for human consumption should be a collection of plant-based foods with flesh—protein—as an addition. The majority of our meals, however, are the exact opposite: a huge lump of animal flesh with plant foods as an afterthought—if they're there at all. Picture a mass of green leaves, a couple of tiny tomatoes, and a lavish calorie-laden creamy dressing, which is a small salad to go with your half a cow.

Nutritionists around the world agree that plant foods have the highest level and widest variety of nutrients, which in turn offer us healthy living. And yet many of us still believe the so-called experts who tell us to eat more protein (specifically, more meat), because that's exactly what we want to believe. I'm not aware of any scientific study that associates increased consumption of plant foods with a high risk of heart disease, diabetes, or cancer. In fact, the opposite is true. Countless scientific studies from around the world associate an increase in meat consumption with many of today's worst diseases, including cancer. The World Cancer Research Fund (WCRF) reviewed 1,013 studies on the relationship between the consumption of red meat and colon (bowel) cancer. The WCRF determined that if you consume more than 500 grams (17.6 ounces) of red meat per week, *not* per meal, your risk of colon cancer rises significantly.

IIIIIIIIIIIIIIIIIIIIIIIIIIIIIIIIIIIIIIIIIIIIIIIIIIIIIIIIIIIIIIIIIIIIIIIIIIIIIIII

TICKELL TIP

No cancer society on the planet tells you to eat
more red meat. On the contrary, all the different cancer
research organizations tell you to eat less. Diets that
advocate a higher consumption of red meat raise your
risk of developing certain cancers. That's a fact.
Stick with fruit, vegetables, fish, and grains.

IIIIIIIIIIIIIIIIIIIIIIIIIIIIIIIIIIIIIIIIIIIIIIIIIIIIIIIIIIIIIIIIIIIIIIIIIIIIIIII

The Okinawans, the longest-living, healthiest people on earth, don't worry about carbs or high-protein diets. ("Carb" isn't a real word in the English dictionary. The word is "carbohydrate"—and "hydrate" is water. "Carb" is an invented word, just like all those invented high-protein, low-carb diets. Muffins and doughnuts and other simple "carbs" have zero water—zero hydrate.) Okinawans eat real food, simple food in moderation, with an emphasis on fruit, vegetables, fish, and grains. It's time we take a page from the Okinawans' playbook and get back to basics—basics and bonuses.

Basic and Bonus

Some nutritionists say there are four food groups and others say there are five, but I say there are only two. I repeat, there are *two* food groups: Basic Foods and Bonus Foods.

Basic Foods are plant foods—vegetables, fruits, grains, nuts, and seeds.

Bonus Foods are not plant foods—red meat, cheese, ice cream, chocolate, fish. The best Bonus Food for human consumption is fish. The Okinawans eat fish every day of their lives—every day through their 80s, 90s, 100s.

But fish has mercury in it! Or so its critics say. Yet the longest-living, healthiest people on earth eat fish every day, and none of my medical colleagues has ever seen a case of fish mercury poisoning! There's probably more heavy metal in a packet of cigarettes than in an entire shark.

The great thing about my program is that I really don't care what you eat. You can actually eat anything you like, even Bonus Foods—in *balance* and *moderation*.

If you live on one type of food to the exclusion of all else, then you're a fanatic. You tend to run out of friends, you never get invited out to dinner, and you run the risk of becoming a social outcast. Where is the balance? Where is the pendulum? If you're a Western-style eater, your pendulum is most likely way over there on the Bonus side. It should really be over toward the Basic side.

While the French are not my favorite example of natural eating, they do have a wonderful phrase, "joie de vivre," which means "joy of living." It's a wonderful phrase to use in conjunction with food. Eating good food is one of the joys of life. Family gatherings, meetings, and celebrations are all enhanced by wonderful food.

If you want to eat meat, go ahead and eat some every now and again. Red meat contains complete protein, iron, and vitamin B_{12}, which is difficult to come by in other foods. So meat can be good for you—again, in moderation, meaning once or twice a week, maybe even three times a week.

What about big pieces of cheese full of saturated animal fat that sticks to the insides of your arteries? The less the better, I say. A good rule of thumb is this: the harder the fat is on your plate, the harder it is in your arteries! But go ahead and eat cheese occasionally. Once or twice a week, certainly no more than three times a week. The same goes for chocolate. A small piece of dark chocolate or two every evening gives a boost of serotonin and endorphins. Simple, right? Easy as apple pie—oh, and that's more apples, less pastry, less fat, less sugar. Generally speaking, simple is always best—especially when it comes to nutrition.

Dr. John's Four Simple Rules of Nutrition

Rule 1: Basic and Bonus

Basic Foods, as we saw earlier, are plant foods. Bonus Foods are not. Err on the side of Basic Foods, and enjoy Bonus Foods in moderation. Swing your dietary pendulum back to Basic Foods.

Rule 2: Two-Thirds, One-Third

If you want to strengthen your immune system and reduce your risk of heart disease, breast cancer, colon cancer, and prostate cancer, two-thirds of the food you eat must come from a plant. In other words, at least two-thirds of your food must come from Basic Foods. Two-thirds Basic, one-third Bonus.

[The Skinny on Protein]

Younger people tend to ask the following: "Well, what about protein? I want big muscles, and you need protein for muscles and strength."

True enough. But meat isn't our only source of protein.

Proteins—there are lots of sources of protein—are made up of building blocks. Have you ever heard of amino acids? I'm guessing you learned about them in school, though you may have forgotten. There are 22 or 23 little building blocks that make up proteins, and nine of these blocks are what we call essential. In other words, the body can't make them. The body can make most of the building blocks, but it can't make those nine; you actually have to eat those building blocks, either in the same meal or within a couple of hours.

The great thing about high-quality protein—meat, fish, eggs, cheese, milk—is that the whole batch of essential amino acids is present in a single food. They're all there; it's that simple. We call foods that contain the nine essential amino acids "complete" protein foods.

Vegetarians have to be careful. They need to put various building blocks together, because most vegetables contain only two or three or four of these essential amino acids—not the whole nine the body requires. To ensure that they're getting all the essential amino acids in the same meal, vegetarians need to eat that with this and this with that. The closest plant food to a "complete" protein is probably soybeans.

(continued . . .)

There's nothing wrong with high-quality proteins. To my
mind, fish is the best high-quality protein. The trouble with a
lot of complete protein foods (especially meat and dairy) is
that they contain a lot of fat as well.

"And what about shellfish?" you ask. "I've heard that it contains cholesterol."

It's interesting, this cholesterol business. About one-quarter
or one-third of the cholesterol in your bloodstream comes
from something you've eaten. The other two-thirds or so is
manufactured by your liver. Why is that? Why does the body
produce cholesterol, if it's something we try not to get much
of? Well, the body needs it to help digestion, to produce sex
hormones, and to produce the protective coating around cell
membranes and nerves.

You definitely need *some* cholesterol; you can't have nil
in your body. The cholesterol produced in the liver is plenty.
However, if you eat a lot of saturated fat (animal fat), your
liver squeezes even more cholesterol into the bloodstream to
help digestion and metabolism. It seems that the more meats,
cheeses, and fatty fast foods you consume, the more cholesterol your liver produces.

Yes, shellfish contains some cholesterol, but listen to this:
If you give a vegetarian pure egg yolks or oysters or prawns
(or anything else with lots of cholesterol), the cholesterol
level in that person's blood doesn't change much. If you give
cholesterol-rich food to a heavy meat and saturated-fat
eater, on the other hand, the blood level of cholesterol goes
up. So it appears to be the combination of saturated animal
fats and cholesterol that is the problem.

You can get away with shellfish some of the time, but you should eat regular fish most of the time when you're looking for good Bonus protein.

The worst meats are obviously lunch meats, hams, and salamis, laden with animal fat that jumps out and almost hits you in the face. And sausages with big lumps of fat—wow, it heads straight for your arteries. Then you come down to your lean lamb and beef—they're not too bad; they contain low amounts of saturated fat if you chop off the visible fat. There's a ton of available iron in red meat as well, which your body needs; and don't forget zinc. As a general rule, pasture-fed beef is more conducive to health than lot-fed beef.

People often say that we should eat more chicken. Yet if you eat chicken with the skin left on, it fills you with—surprise!— more saturated fat than lamb or beef. Skinless chicken, on the other hand, contains less saturated fat than red meat.

When it comes to high-quality protein, fish is still the clear winner. For one thing, it contains way more omega-3 fatty acids (important for overall health) than red meat or chicken. *Way* more.

Lots of people keep pushing high-protein eating regimens, but let's face it: the body doesn't need as much protein as it matures into middle age and beyond. Besides, I keep going back to the races of people who live a long time and have little cancer, heart disease, or arthritis. My heroes, the Okinawans, for example. These folks eat a vast range of plant foods along with some protein and little animal fat.

For weight loss, diet proponents such as Dr. Atkins, Dr. Dukan, and the Paleo pals have been trying to convince us

(continued . . .)

that high-animal protein, high-fat diets work and are safe.
One thing I know for sure is that the great majority of American diet gurus have never gone to a country that has no
fat people and watched them eat. I'll say it again—the diet
of those lean and healthy people consists of a vast range
of plant foods, with *some* protein (including plenty of fish)
and very little animal fat. What they forget to tell you is that
high-protein diets mean high fat. Excess protein puts a strain
on your kidneys as we age and leeches calcium out of your
bones.

Sure, a high-protein, high-fat, and low-carb diet produces
weight loss, but no greater weight loss than a lower-protein
diet. And even if you're among the 5 percent of Western-style
dieters who succeed, weight loss isn't everything. The fact
remains that eating food high in fat and protein over a long
period of time increases the risk of cancer, the biggest health
problem in the Western world today. We can fix lots of broken
hearts, but fixing cancer is far more difficult. And what about
three years down the road for those high-protein dieters?
Have they kept the weight off?

Still not convinced? Well, in Australia, where I'm from, the
Commonwealth Scientific and Industrial Research Organization tried to prove that a diet high in protein produced more
weight loss than a lower-protein diet. They failed miserably.
Their research showed that, over 12 weeks, the people in the
high-protein group lost only 1.5 pounds more than the people
in the low-protein group. And they lost an average of only 15
pounds over the 12-week trial. Through my meal plan, people
can lose that amount in 6 weeks, not 12.

Maybe you'll go into a hotel or restaurant tonight and tell the waiter that Dr. John said you could have a Bonus Food, so you order steak. You order it medium-rare, nice and juicy. When the plate comes, however, you see that the kitchen screwed up the rule: they gave you more than two-thirds Bonus Foods and less than one-third Basic Foods. Ironically, many restaurants charge extra for good plant sides.

Compare this to how the Okinawans eat. Their plates are covered with vegetables, along with some rice and a small portion of flesh, usually either fish or chicken. They have the rule right—two-thirds Basic, one-third Bonus.

Rule 3: HI Instead of GI

After you eat carbohydrates, your blood sugar level—literally the level of glucose in your bloodstream—goes up. You've probably heard of the glycemic index, or GI, which is a measure of how quickly this spike occurs. Because different foods affect blood sugar differently, the glycemic index estimates how much a gram of carbohydrate raises a person's glucose level, relative to the consumption of pure glucose. Foods with carbohydrates that break down slowly and release glucose gradually into the bloodstream tend to have a low GI. Conversely, foods with carbohydrates that break down quickly during digestion and release glucose rapidly into the bloodstream tend to have a high GI.

Vegetables and fruits, as we all know, are the best foods on earth. But did you know they're mainly all carbohydrates? Vegetables have a lower GI than fruits, however, because they release glucose slowly into the bloodstream. Okinawans rely heavily on these carbohydrates. As a result, they're lean and energetic and have a very low risk of heart disease and cancer. Why would you want to do anything different?

Unless you're a diabetic, you don't need to bother about the glycemic index. It often makes people freak out, because they see a number higher than 45 or 55 or whatever. For a bit of a laugh, take a look at these GI ratings for literally the same foods, based on two recent wildly popular diets.

	Atkins Diet	South Beach Diet
Brown Rice	55	79
Banana	52	89
Watermelon	72	103
Baked Potato	85	158
Sweet Potato	54	63
Chickpeas	33	47
White Bread	70	101

Confused? Good. So am I.

A food's GI rating is irrelevant, as long as you're eating foods that have a low HI index. What's that? It's an index I invented to measure "human interference." In other words, my HI index measures how badly human beings have messed with the food or drink in front of you!

Think about a potato. Under most circumstances, a potato is good, wholesome food. The Okinawans have been relying on sweet potatoes for hundreds of years. But when we Americans live on potatoes, we slice each one into 45 fries! We increase the surface area hundreds of times, cover the slices in salt, and dump them in hot fat. We interfere with the potato, which makes the health consequences disastrous. A potato has an HI rating of 0. French fries, on the other hand, have an HI rating of at least 6. (We'll talk more about how to calculate a food's HI rating in chapter 6.)

Another example is an apple. We pick beautiful, natural apples in the orchard. There's no human interference. But then we take them home. We slice them, dice them, and cook them. And then we add pastry. We add all kinds of fat, sugar, and salt. And *then* we add cream or ice cream, which is about 99.99 percent calories! More human interference, and even more disastrous health consequences.

The standard American diet consists overwhelmingly of processed and highly refined foods—foods with incredibly high HI levels and calorie content. Right now, you're probably thinking about your favorite muffin. "I *love* my morning muffin," you say. That's fine. I don't want to take away your muffin. I just want you to have one or two bites and leave the rest. "But, Doctor, my muffin cost four dollars. I can't *waste* part of it." Well, but it's four dollars either way—eaten entirely or nibbled on. In the meantime, you're continuing to bring on illness and disease earlier and earlier in life. Bottom line—do you want those excess calories to go to waste or to your waist?

Generally speaking, the more refined a product is—that is, the higher its human interference quotient—the quicker it enters the bloodstream, forcing your pancreas to produce insulin. Many people develop adult onset diabetes because of this breakdown in the system. More and more now, it's happening in our children as well! Adult-onset diabetes has become childhood-onset diabetes. Whose fault is that? Even though my mother used to tell me, "Eat all the food on your plate," I know for certain she wouldn't tell me that today, with the "supersize" servings we dish up today.

It's fairly obvious that the refining of food—the increase of human interference—has a lot to answer for, because the countries with the most refined foods have easily the largest number of diabetics, by a long way.

|||||||||||||||||||||||||||||||||||||||||||||||||||||||||||||||||||||||||||||||||

TICKELL TIP

Parents and grandparents are the best
role models for their children and grandchildren.
Children don't usually do what you *tell* them to do. They
do what you *do*. They copy. Your children have an
80 percent chance of ending up like you or your partner.
Make sure you set a good example. While you're Loving,
Laughing, and Eating your way to 100, you're also
helping your kids learn to do the same.

|||||||||||||||||||||||||||||||||||||||||||||||||||||||||||||||||||||||||||||||||

I've already told you that counting calories doesn't work long-term. But *comparing* calories does work—that is, comparing the calories of various meals as a way to understand that eating good, low-HI food is health-conducive and eating bad, high-HI food is a disaster.

Compare a takeaway meal and a healthy meal:

> A big burger with medium fries and a milkshake or soda comes in at around 1,000 calories. A three-piece meal of fried chicken plus a bag of chips and a drink is more than 1,000 calories.

> A bowl of salad and a slice of multigrain bread or toast with a few drops of olive oil, on the other hand, is about 300 calories. Baked beans and tomato on toast is about 220 calories. A bowl of vegetable soup and a slice of soy and linseed toast is 220 calories.

What's the difference? About 700 to 800 calories a day, or more than 70 pounds per year, between takeout and a healthier alternative.

Another comparison:

> A large order of fries is about 400 calories.
>
> A medium baked potato with sour cream is 150 calories (less with low-fat sour cream).
>
> A scoop of mashed potato made with milk is 40 calories.

How about your snacks?

> A single-serve packet of salt and vinegar potato chips is approximately 500 calories.
>
> A slice of cheesecake contains about 380 calories.
>
> A doughnut contains about 340 calories.
>
> A muffin comes in at about 220 calories.
>
> A can of Coke alone has 160 calories!

In comparison, look at these healthy snack options:

> A mandarin orange has only about 30 calories.
>
> A slice of crisp bread with tomato has about 40 calories.
>
> A handful of almonds has about 80 calories.
>
> A couple of celery sticks with hummus dip add only about 40 calories.
>
> A generous dollop of low-fat yogurt (3.5 ounces) is about 90 calories.

You getting the point yet? An extra 160 calories per day, over a year, can add up to 16 pounds of weight. (Remember that a pound of fat equals 3,500 calories.)

[Fat]

Most people consider fat the enemy, but not all fat is out to get us. People on a diet often try to limit their fat intake. Why? Because fat contains more calories per ounce than carbohydrates and proteins. Sounds sensible, right? Well, yes and no.

All fats and oils have the same number of calories, but *good* fats—particularly monounsaturated fats (more on them below)—help the body absorb nutrients, especially vitamins, and they trigger positive responses for cell membranes. They help your skin, they help manage your mood, and they're an important source of energy. And science agrees that omega-3 gives the immune system a boost.

Let's look at the range of fats found in foods.

In our society, the most commonly eaten fat (most "popular" fat) is *saturated fat*. Animal fat is the most common saturated fat. Most scientists agree on the association between the consumption of saturated fat and the tragically high level of heart attacks in this country. Less is better—it's obvious that the longest-living people on earth eat little saturated fat.

Some plant fats and plant oils are primarily saturated as well. Coconut oil, palm oil, and cocoa butter, for example, can act on the body like animal fats, though in their natural state a little is okay.

Unsaturated fat is another popular fat. Unlike saturated fat, which is solid and sticky and hard to break down, unsaturated fat is oily and liquid and easily absorbed. Unsaturated fats are common in fish oils, vegetable oils (such as those pressed from sunflower seeds, olives, and avocados), wild-caught fish, and organic eggs.

Unsaturated fat has two subtypes: monounsaturated fat and polyunsaturated fat.

Monounsaturated fat, favored throughout the Mediterranean, is found in extra-virgin olive oil, macadamia nuts, and avocados. This is the safest kind of fat. Enjoy it!

Most plant oils and fish oils are *polyunsaturated.* Like monounsaturated fats, these are liquid at room temperature—that is, they don't stick—so they move through your arteries and tissues. Omega-3 and omega-6 oils fall into this category. Both are beneficial, though the levels have gotten way out of balance in recent times. We need more 3s and fewer 6s (the latter found, for example, in vegetable oils and chicken). So opt for more fish oil, olive oil, and flaxseed oil—the prime sources of omega-3s.

Skip the *trans fat* entirely. It's made by transforming unsaturated vegetable fat into saturated fat through the process of hydrogenation. The result is a complete disaster. This immune-system wrecker hides in such things as cookies, cakes, pastries, doughnuts, muffins, margarine, potato chips, crackers, and most fried foods. Trans fat decreases good cholesterol, increases bad cholesterol, and can heighten the risk of cancer and heart disease.

Rule 4: The Rule of 15

Among these four rules, the Rule of 15 has the greatest influence on changing people's attitudes about food. Not only does my favorite rule alter your focus, and not only will you begin to have more energy and eat less of the crap foods as the rule becomes second nature, but you're likely to reduce your risk of potentially preventable cancers by a significant margin. The largely preventable cancers include breast, bowel, prostate, and lung. Cancers of the brain, pancreas, and ovaries are more accurately categorized as "bad luck" cancers, although ovarian cancer does seem to be less common in women who are regularly active and eat Basic Foods more than Bonus Foods.

How can I make the claim that breast, bowel, prostate, and lung cancers are potentially preventable? Because of the numbers. As we saw in an earlier chapter, in the islands of Okinawa it is stated that 6 in 100,000 women die from breast cancer, according to the Okinawan Centenarian Study and other scientific research. In the United States, conversely, the number is 33 in 100,000.

Some argue that this difference is due to genetics. Yet when these low-risk folks migrate to the so-called civilized Western world, their risks become similar to ours within a couple of generations.

So what *is* the Rule of 15? It asks merely that you try to eat 15 or more bits and pieces of plant variety food every day. It's no big deal and fairly simple to do. Notice that I didn't use the word "vegetables." I wrote "plant variety." This means vegetables, yes—but also fruits, grains, nuts, and seeds. And notice that I said "bits and pieces," not "huge amounts" of each. Easy, right? If my 13-year-old daughter could do it—and she did—you can too.

I asked in the preceding paragraph that you "try" to follow the Rule of 15. That's an overused phrase, and I should have avoided it. Instead, I'll turn it into a lesson.

Last week, a guy said to me proudly, "I tried to go to the gym three times last week."

I responded, "You tried? Did you go or not?"

"Ah, well, not really," he said.

Forget the word "try" when it comes to you managing you. Either you do it or you don't.

All you have to do to follow this rule is keep a bowl or plate of five or six different vegetables on your counter or in your refrigerator. In addition, buy some unsalted nuts, olives, dates, and seed mix for the occasional snacks. Trust me, if you surround yourself with these foods, you will eat them.

||||||||||||||||||||||||||||||||||||||||||||||||||||||||||||||||||||||||||||||||||

TICKELL TIP

Cut up various fruits into bite-size chunks, put them in
a bowl or on a platter, and pop it into the refrigerator.
Your fridge should have a fresh-fruit platter in it
100 percent of the time. I call this the FP100. "My
children won't eat fruit!" you say. Yes, they will, if you
cut it up into bite-size chunks. Making an FP100 takes
approximately five to seven minutes each day. This
is one of the *best* secrets from Down Under. It was
invented by my wife (and best friend), Sue, who's in her
60s—and (no coincidence here) is the same weight she
was before she gave birth to our five children.
Do it. No excuses.

||||||||||||||||||||||||||||||||||||||||||||||||||||||||||||||||||||||||||||||||||

Here's a list of solid foods and liquids I regularly eat and drink to achieve the all-important variety of foods the human body needs. (In fact, it's a list of what I ate yesterday!)

Banana	Soy and linseed bread
Carrot	Sardines
Strawberries	Yogurt
Coffee	Olives
Brussels sprouts	Soy milk
Passion fruit	Alfalfa sprouts
Grapes	Avocado
Lamb chop	Almonds
Spring onions	Prunes
Mandarin orange	Tomato
Corn	Beets
Raspberries	Soybeans
Water	Red wine

As you can see, 19 are Basic Foods (20, if you count red wine!). And I did *not* eat a whole avocado, a whole carrot, 20 strawberries, and multiple lamb chops. The trick is to eat just small amounts. Twenty-six different types of food and drink—most of them plant-based. You don't need to eat all of these, but after a few days you'll begin to broaden your horizons.

Remember, you can't count refined or processed foods in applying the Rule of 15. *Refined products don't count!* White bread doesn't count. Table sugar doesn't count. Coco Pops don't count.

Why not? If you can't tell me why not by now, read on . . .

Let's take a look at a normal day to illustrate how easy it is to satisfy the Rule of 15. This is a typical example of Sue's breakfast every morning:

½ grapefruit	Small piece of orange
2 prunes	Small piece of watermelon
½ passion fruit	Small piece of cantaloupe
1 date	Slice of kiwi
1 dried apricot	6 almonds
1 strawberry	6 pistachios
Small piece of pineapple	Cup of tea

Most of these come from the FP100 that lives in our refrigerator. It takes four minutes a day to cut up the fruit into bite-size chunks. The kids *love* it. The grandkids *love* it.

Admittedly, some people think that Sue's routine is a bit over-the-top, but you could easily eat five or six fruit portions for breakfast, along with a few oats and maybe a dab of yogurt. (Again, these are not five or six *whole* fruits. A single fruit lacks the variety we want, so small bits of multiple fruits are better.)

In fact, when it comes to breakfast, variety is the name of the game. Fruits and whole grains and nuts are great in partnership, and—if you're feeling adventurous and willing to learn from our Okinawan brethren—you can even incorporate small amounts of fish, beans, and rice. If you're not willing to go the whole hog, so to speak, you should at least keep a bowl of cut fruit in your refrigerator at all times. This is good advice regardless. Depending on the season, you might be able to throw in five, six, even eight different types of fruits, including fresh berries, which makes for a wonderful variety of healthy and delicious food.

Lunch could then include a piece of soy and pumpkin-seed bread, and—if you're eating out—a wide selection from the salad bar (four, five, or six bits and pieces of plant, along with some cheese or a small bit of tuna or salmon). If you're at home, baked beans and tomato on soy and linseed bread gives you another four. Another, easier option: simply crack open a can of vegetable soup—one without a lot of salt or other additives.

Already, you're at least at 10 out of 15. Grab a few unsalted nuts or olives or dates throughout the day and you're almost there. $6 + 4 + 2 = 12$.

For dinner, eat a small piece of fish, turkey, or lean meat and at least three vegetables, if not four or five. "But we usually have only one or two," you might argue. Well, your grandmother, I'm sure, used to cook five types of vegetables every night. It's not impossible. Sue, when she's cooking at home, does at least eight or ten vegetables, cooking them as a single batch. She says it takes the same amount of time as doing a huge pile of one or two vegetables. And truly, both kids and dinner guests love the array. Many of our families today are so busy during the day that they need to do a quickie meal, which usually means pasta with sauces, creams, or something heated up in the microwave—something quick! The good news is that vegetables can be brought to the table very quickly!

TICKELL TIP

Another great Japanese phrase is *Hara hachi bu*,
which means, "Eat until you are 80 percent full."
Eat less food and eat more slowly.
There's a 20-minute delay between when your
stomach is nearly full and when your brain receives
that message and knows what's happening. Slow down.
Really taste your food. Savor it.

Nuchi gusui is a Japanese phrase meaning, "May your food and your lifestyle heal." Each time you begin to stuff your face with doughnuts, brownies, or burgers, ask yourself this simple question: Is this food healing or hurting me?

Are your cheeseburgers and fries healing you or hurting you? And what about those crazy high-protein diets, which the World Cancer Research Fund tells us increase our risk of cancer? Are the foods recommended by those diets healing you or hurting you?

If a food heals you, eat it. If it hurts you, skip it. Maybe take a bite or two, then leave the rest on the plate. Try visualizing what kind of damage it would do to your insides. That will help you walk away. It's totally your call. It's your choice. It's your health. It's your life.

What Went Wrong with the Western Way?	
Activity	We don't move.
Coping	Life is too complex.
Eating	Human interference—we take good food and wreck it. We oversize our servings, which makes for oversize people. We get stuck in a rut: lack of food variety becomes boring. We forget the Basic Foods and replace them with *Bonus* Foods.

PART TWO

Skills to Love, Laugh, and Eat

━━

Chapter 4

Activity Skills

Having studied patterns of human behavior for three decades, I took the strategy most associated with success in other fields of human endeavor and applied it to weight loss. This strategy has been tested over and over again, and the proof has been confirmed. It works, and in my mind it's the only way to lose weight and keep it off for *long-term* success.

This foolproof method is the so-called stepped approach: two steps forward and one step back. In the case of weight loss, the best approach is a slight variant: three steps forward and two steps back.

I call my variation of the stepped approach the Switch On, Then Hold approach.

When an athlete achieves his or her personal best, a period of underperformance often follows. An athlete doesn't continue to perform at the same peak level, but instead consolidates the training and effort that made the personal best possible. After this brief period of consolidation, he or she can move on to the next level of achievement. This "stepping" is necessary because the limit of human endurance, or sustained human excellence, is 21 days. I'll say it again: the limit of human endurance, of doing something full on, is 21 days.

Diets fail for the same reason that athletes can't sustain a peak continuously. People on a diet think they can just keep on doing it, with the same level of success and commitment they started out with. Inevitably, they falter—usually within the first three weeks. Then they plateau. Then they give up and go back to their old ways, at least for a time. The weight comes off, the weight goes back on—off, on—off, on. Ad infinitum. It just doesn't work.

The Switch On, Then Hold approach is the most sensible way I know of to achieve your personal best. It succeeds because it recognizes and takes into account our human endurance limitations.

And the best part is that you don't need to be fanatical about exercise.

Broadly speaking, there are three levels of activity:

a. Fanatical
b. Moderate
c. Zero (slob)

Personally, I think B is a great choice. I trust that you chose B as well. If you chose A, we'll see you at the next Olympic Games. However, if you're over the age of 35 and you chose A, be very careful, because it might kill you.

It's okay not to exercise every day. But it's an excellent idea to be active in some way every day. That's why the Activity section grounds my ACE program.

[**Medical Disclaimer**]

Many experts say that you *must* get checked by a doctor or physician before you start any exercise program. Question: Do Asian villagers check with their doctor before they walk a mile to get some water or hike through the hills to tend their animals? No, they don't, because there is no doctor.

Do you check with your doctor before you walk to the bus stop or the train station? Probably not.

Nevertheless, it is a medical practice and a legal necessity to say to you that you *must* have a medical checkup before you commence an exercise program. Your doctor may think it's a waste of time and you may think it's a waste of money, but that's what's necessary in our world today.

The Switch On, Then Hold approach is specifically designed to give you a bit of a break from whatever formal exercises you choose to undertake.

I want you to think about what's good for you, and then get into this moving thing regularly. To think and to be aware—and then to act. Take the stairs next time instead of the elevator. Walk to the corner store to pick up the newspaper or milk. Take your dog for a walk. Don't just watch your kids at play; join them. Become a child again at the park and crawl under the table to pick up that stray piece of paper. Or take a stroll with your partner after dinner while you have a chat. You'll start to love what happens when activity becomes a part of you.

Activity Skills

Activity starts with the first step. Then it continues one step at a time. A cliché, for sure. But clichés are clichés for a reason: they're true. When you get active, or when you laugh, or when you love, your body produces endorphins, which are opioid chemicals that make you feel incredible. They give you a natural high. Once you get the body going, it starts to respond by releasing more of these powerful endorphins, which make you feel better and better.

Walking is great, especially if you're carrying some pudding around your waist or thighs. Most of us travel to work on wheels—not bicycle wheels, but car wheels or bus wheels. Some of us travel on train tracks. But few of us walk or cycle to work. And once we get to work, we sit around for hours at a time, in front of computers.

And how about school? Kids sit around there too, in front of computers. And before and after school, kids stare at television sets and computer screens and smartphones.

Walking is the centerpiece of the Activity section of my ACE program. Which is why I want you to walk four or five days a week for 25 minutes. Or six days a week for 20 minutes. I don't care which; it's entirely your choice.

The point is to walk briskly enough that you're lightly puffing. If you want to walk with someone else, that's fine. If you prefer, do it by yourself—that's fine too. If you want to walk fewer than four days per week, forget it.

SBW: Strong(er) Is Better Than Weak

Once you hit your 30s, muscle strength starts to deteriorate slowly—at first. It then deteriorates more rapidly. As a result, most mature Westerners are weak.

[How Are You Traveling?]

Traveling is no excuse for slacking off on activity. Make a point of checking into a hotel located by a park or a beach. A swimming pool is also very handy. Use your briefcase as a hand-weight or unpack half your clothes and use the partially emptied bag as a hand-weight (instead of using a dumbbell). Push-ups, triceps work using a chair, and abdominal tightening are easy—you don't need a gym for those exercises.

Hotel fire escapes are great for multiple uses: if there's a fire you go down the stairs, and when there's no fire you go up the stairs! What I do is this. First, I check that the fire escape door will open from inside the stairwell so that I can get back into the building. Then I go down a few flights of stairs as a warm-up before walking up the stairs. (Don't do this if you're not relatively fit.) Then I catch the elevator down and walk up the stairs again. (Personally, I don't keep walking *down* the stairs because it bothers my back, but you can certainly walk down as well if you wish.) Down, up, down, up—I keep doing this until I've had enough, but not until I'm exhausted. I'm sure the hotel maids think I'm crazy!

Even when I'm not in a hotel, I still aim to climb at least 200 stairs each day, as I noted earlier. That's not as rigorous as it sounds. Remember, it's 20 times 10 or 10 times 20 spread throughout the day. The handy thing is, there are stairs everywhere. (Again, don't start off at 200 stairs the first day. Work up to that amount over the course of many weeks.)

I've already mentioned the 600 muscles and 180 joints in your body. If your muscles are reasonably strong, they help take the strain off your joints, a collaboration that also gives you more energy. Muscles also burn a lot more calories than fat does—so having good, well-toned muscles actually helps with weight loss. You don't need huge muscles. You just need strong, well-toned muscles.

In her mid-40s, my lovely wife, Sue, gave birth to our fifth child, a bouncing baby boy. He is now 21! A 14-year gap between child number four and child number five is not great for anyone's body. But turning a negative into a positive is Sue's specialty. Well, that and her college degree in physical education. Some trainers have done a six-week course in fitness, while Sue's education was four years. She designed a simple program to tone, firm, and strengthen her muscles in all the right spots.

"I'm a busy person," she reminded me, "with five kids and eight grandchildren, and I work as well. If I can spend a few minutes four or five times a week exercising my bottom, arms, and tummy, so can anyone."

The places in which we typically accumulate excesses of fat are our bottoms, arms, and tummies, so why not give them something positive to do each day? If we sit around, eating and drinking additional calories, those body parts simply conform to our peculiar way of degenerating.

Sue's program focuses on these three specific areas, and it works well for female and male bottoms, arms, and tummies. Sue is BAT Woman—Bottom, Arms, Tummy. The program's beauty lies in its simplicity. All you need is a room, a pair of light hand-weights, and a desire to reshape your body. Combine these exercises with your four or five or six walks each week, gradually increasing the toning activity sets and varying the repetitions as you progress.

Here's an example of how to set up your own program, utilizing my Switch On, Then Hold approach.

	Sets	Repetitions
Week 1	1	6
Week 2	1	8
Week 3	1	10
Week 4 *Entirely up to you.*		
Week 5 *Also entirely up to you.*		
Week 6	2	6
Week 7	2	8
Week 8	2	10
Week 9 *No worries.*		
Week 10 *You're doing great.*		
Week 11	2	6
Week 12	2	8
Week 13	2	10

Bottom, Arms, and Tummy (BAT Exercises)

As we mature throughout our lives, some people excuse all sorts of failings by saying, "Well, we are all getting older, aren't we?" I guess there is some truth to that, but my response is this—you can grow old gracefully, or you can fight it every inch of the way!

Sue is an excellent example of the latter approach, though she's not really fighting. She simply does what she's always done: she looks after her mind and body.

You might reply, "Yes, but I'm too old. I'm too rusty [or stiff or arthritic] to do these things." Well, Sue is 65 and bore five children, and she's a terrific personal trainer. Her mature clients are in their 70s and 80s, so we'll accept your excuse only if you're in your 90s or 100s.

Bottom

Bridge

Lie on your back with your knees bent and your feet slightly apart.
Rest your arms at your side. Push your hips upward, bottom off
the floor, tightening your bottom. Hold for two or three seconds,
then lower your bottom back to the floor.

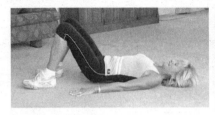
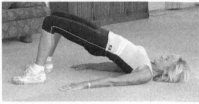

Side Leg Lifts

Lie on your right side, resting your body weight on your elbow.
Bend your right leg to a comfortable angle and keep your left
leg straight. Slowly raise your left leg to just above hip level.
Gently return your left leg to the starting position. Repeat on
the other side.

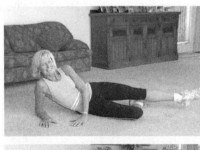
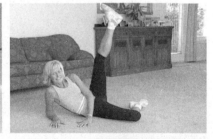
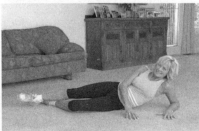
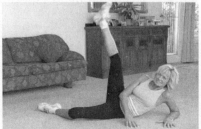

Leg Extensions

Kneel on all fours, keeping your back straight. Bring your left knee slightly forward and then extend your left leg straight back. Immediately repeat with your right leg.

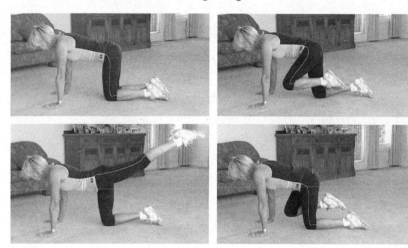

Arms

Biceps

Stand with your right foot slightly ahead of your left, keeping your back straight. Hold the hand-weight in your right hand (palm facing forward). Women, start with a hand-weight of approximately five pounds. Men, start with an eight-pound weight. Keep your right elbow in toward the body. Slowly curl the hand-weight forward and up toward your right shoulder; then lower the hand-weight. After the required repetitions, repeat with your left arm.

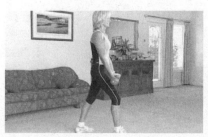 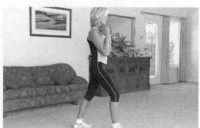

Triceps

Sit on a chair with your knees bent at a 90-degree angle and your feet flat. Curl your fingers around the front of the seat for support. Slide your bottom forward and off the edge, keeping it close to the seat. Point your elbows back and in. Lower and then lift yourself with your arms, keeping your back straight. (Beginner dips are done with knees bent. As you progress, straighten your legs more.)

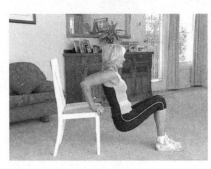 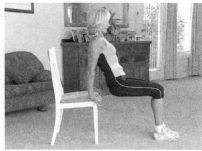

Shoulders

Stand with your feet shoulder-width apart. Keep your back straight and your arms in front of you. Hold the hand-weights with your palms facing you. With your elbows bent slightly, bring the weights straight up to your chin. Your forearms should be parallel to the floor, as if you were going to pull yourself out of a swimming pool. Slowly lower the weights back to the starting position.

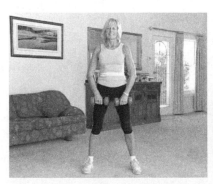 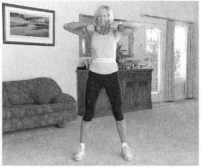

Tummy

For all three crunches—up, across, and side-to-side—lie on your
back with your legs bent and your feet shoulder-width apart.

Up

Place your hands, palms down, on your thighs. Slide your hands up
toward your knees, lifting your head and shoulders slightly off the
floor. Your lower back should remain firmly on the floor.

Across

Reach your left hand across to your right knee and then your right
hand across to your left knee, again lifting your head and shoulders
slightly off the floor. Your lower back should remain firmly on the floor.

Side-to-Side

Reach your left hand to the outside of your left ankle and then
your right hand to the outside of your right ankle. Your lower back
should remain firmly on the floor.

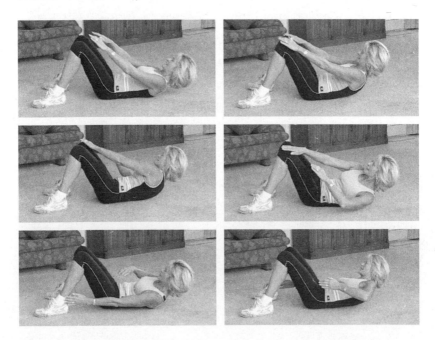

Bonus BATs: Boobs and Pecs

Flies

Lie on your back with your legs bent and your feet on the floor, slightly apart. Hold the hand-weights straight above your chest. Your palms should face each other and your elbows should be bent. Gently lower your arms out and down until your upper arms reach the floor. Return the weights to the starting position.

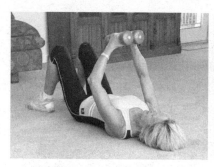 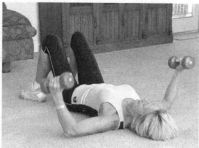

Push-Up A

Face a wall, standing about three shoe lengths from it, your feet flat and almost together. Place your hands flat against the wall, shoulder-width apart. Keep your body and legs in a straight line and bend your elbows as you lower yourself toward the wall. Gently push back to the starting position.

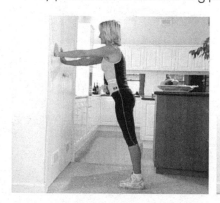 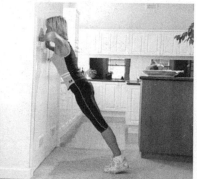

Push-Up B

Repeat the steps of Push-Up A, but use a waist-high bench instead of a wall.

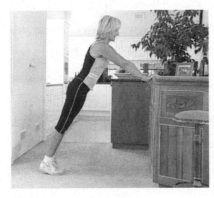 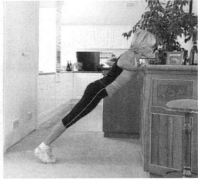

Push-Up C

Kneel on all fours. Keep your hands shoulder-width apart directly below your shoulders and your knees close together. Bend your elbows and gently lower your torso toward the floor, while maintaining the straight position from your head to your bottom. Push up by straightening your arms.

Men, when you get good at push-ups off your knees, try a couple of push-ups off your feet.

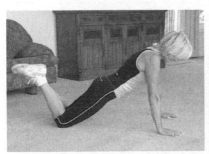 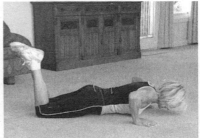

OUMs: Other Useful Movements

Some people call these stretches, but I prefer other useful movements, or OUMs, largely because I am, despite my best efforts to the contrary, a type A person at work, and I rarely have 30 minutes to stretch. Still, flexibility is crucial, especially if you tend to get back and/or neck pain. A couple of minutes' stretching and flexibility work will give you a huge payback.

Do some OUMs before or after your walk, and include some neck and back movements regularly, especially if you have an office job or drive a car for long periods of time.

My daughters, Anna and Amanda, are both highly qualified physiotherapists, and they helped me put together a list of OUMs.

Let's move down the body, from head to foot, and do a few useful movements.

Do the OUMs just *once* in each session. Some are *limbering* movements or warm-ups, and the others are *holds,* which means you hold in one position for around 10 seconds. We'll call them L movements and H movements.

OUMs relate to the following body bits:

L	H
Neck	Chest
Shoulders	Hamstrings
Sides	Thighs/Quads
Back	Calves
Feet	

OUM Limbering Exercises

Neck

Stand with your feet apart and your arms at your sides. Tilt your head slowly to your right side, bringing your right ear toward your right shoulder. Then slowly tilt your head toward your left side, bringing your left ear toward your left shoulder. Return your head to a straight position. Repeat three times. Turn your head to the right, looking beyond your right shoulder; then slowly turn your head to the other side. Repeat three times.

Easy does it. Don't jerk your head around, and absolutely positively do *not* rotate your neck in complete circles.

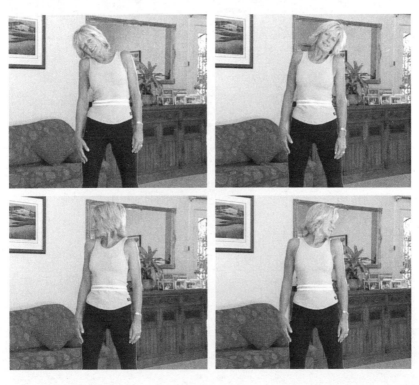

Shoulders

Stand with your feet apart and your arms at your sides. Hunch your shoulders slightly forward, then roll them gently upward. Pull your shoulders back firmly before relaxing them down to a natural resting position. Repeat three times.

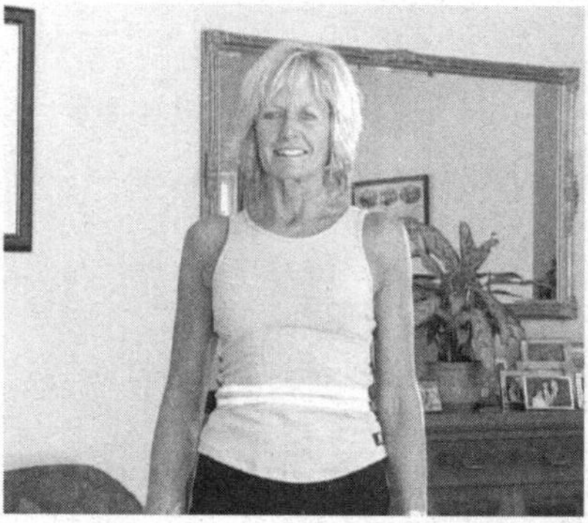

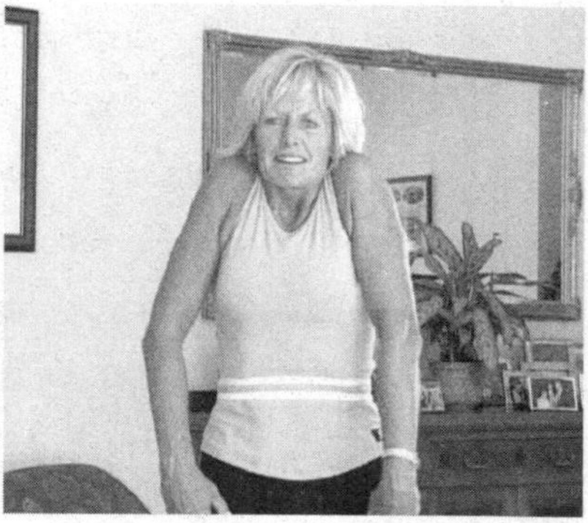

TICKELL TIP

Sue tells me it's good to mix up the L movements and the H movements rather than doing all the holds in a row.

Sides

Stand with your feet shoulder-width apart and your arms hanging relaxed at your sides. Lift your right arm slowly out and up from your side, keeping it relaxed but almost straight. Slide your left arm down your left leg, gently reaching your right arm high above your head. Slowly bring both arms back to your sides. Repeat on the other side. Stretch your right and left sides three times each.

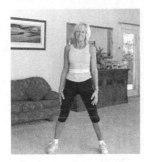 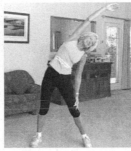 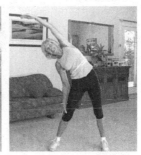

Back

Stand facing away from a wall. Keep your feet flat and legs apart, roughly a shoe length from the wall. Slowly rotate your torso to your right, toward the wall, with both hands reaching for it. Gently turn your torso back and reach to your left, again toward the wall, with both hands reaching for it. Repeat three times.

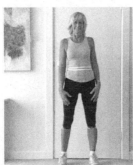 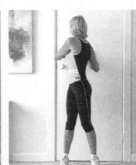 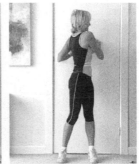

Feet

Hold on to the back of a chair for balance. Stand on your left leg
and slowly circle your right foot five times in one direction. Then
circle the same foot five times in the other direction. Now stand on
your right leg and repeat the movements with your left foot.

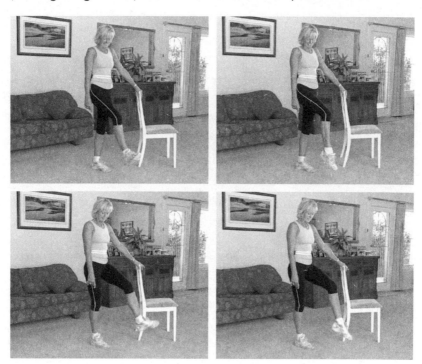

OUM Hold Exercises

Chest

Stand in a doorway with your body straight and your feet almost together. Bend your arms at the elbows and raise your arms so that your upper arms are perpendicular to the floor and your palms are flat against the door frame. Step slowly forward with one leg until your shoulders are back. You'll start to feel your chest stretch. Hold this position for 10 seconds. After returning to the starting position, step forward with the other leg and hold.

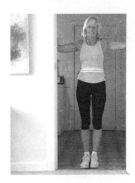
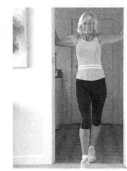
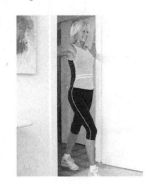

Hamstrings

Stand behind a chair, holding the top of the chair's back with both hands. Place one foot well in front of the other, moving it under the chair. Slowly bend your back leg at the knee and press back into a "sitting" position, while flexing the foot in front of you. Hold for 10 seconds, then repeat on the other side.

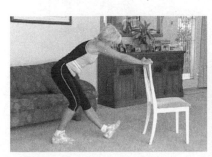
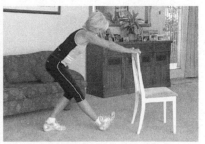

Thighs/Quads

Stand behind a chair, holding the top of the chair's back with your right hand. Bend your left leg at the knee and, with your left hand, pull it up so that your left foot approaches your buttocks or until you feel your leg muscle stretch. Hold for 10 seconds. Bring your left foot down and repeat with your right leg.

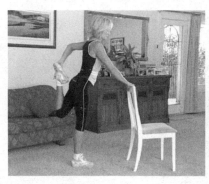 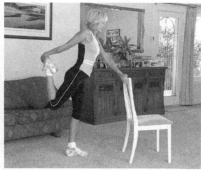

Calves

Stand behind a chair, holding the top of the chair's back with both hands. Place one foot well in front of the other, with your feet lined up. Bend your front leg while keeping your back leg straight, heel on the floor. Gently press forward until you feel your calf muscle stretch. Hold for 10 seconds. Repeat with your other leg.

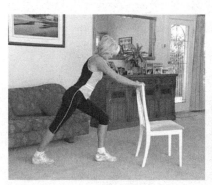 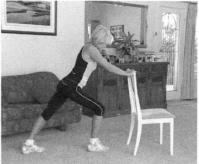

|||||||||||||||||||||||||||||||||||||||||||||||||||||||||||||||||||||||||||||||||

TICKELL TIP

Activity requires energy, which burns calories. If you

stay active, here's what you burn doing these things:

Sleeping: 40–60 calories per hour

Sitting: 60–100 calories per hour

Walking: 200–300 calories per hour

Cycling: 300–500 calories per hour

Swimming: 400–600 calories per hour

Running: 600–1,000 calories per hour

Sex (on top): 400 calories per hour (5 minutes = 33 calories)

Sex (on your back): 0–200 calories per hour

Cooking: 100–200 calories per hour

(Tasting while you cook, however,

will add 200 calories per hour.)

Do *some* activity five days a week. Over a year, the fat

will perform a disappearing act. Check these activity

options out, with the expected weight loss for each

(assuming five days a week of that particular activity):

30-minute walk: 7–10 pounds expected weight loss in one year

30-minute bike ride: 7–15 pounds expected weight loss in one year

30-minute swim: 15–20 pounds expected weight loss in one year

30-minute run: 15–25 pounds expected weight loss in one year

|||||||||||||||||||||||||||||||||||||||||||||||||||||||||||||||||||||||||||||||||

The Numbers Game

For a start, let's not worry about dropping off pounds. Focus instead on adding up numbers.

Every point you tally in the ACE program is known as a Liv-ing*life* point. The idea is to score around 72 of these Living*life* points during Switch On weeks. (If you're bothered about keeping score, that aversion probably started at school, with grades—As and Bs and all that stuff.) During the Hold weeks, rack up as many points as you want, but ideally your goal should still be around 72 Living*life* points.

While other diet programs want you to count carbs, calories, or kangaroos, my ACE program wants you to earn points for laughing and for touching your toes. That's right. You actually get points for hugging your kids and your loved ones—and for feeling ready, willing, and able.

Give yourself two points each time you walk. Then give yourself a point for your BAT and OUM exercises. A point, too, for every one of Four Simple Rules of Nutrition that you follow (e.g., the Two-Thirds, One-Third Rule and the Rule of 15). Same goes for every single thing you do from my Relaxation List (which you'll learn more about in the next chapter, titled "Coping Skills.") Yes, you can score points in the game of life for relaxing!

What's this got to do with losing weight?

Everything!

Ask yourself these questions every day:

> **Did I do my walk today?**
>
> **Did I do my toning work today?**
>
> **Did I do my OUMs today?**
>
> **Did I do my coping work today?**
>
> **Did I do my meal plan today?**

Sound like hard work? No, it's easy. Just do it.

|||||||||||||||||||||||||||||||||||||||||||||||||||||||||||||||||||||||||||||||||||||||||||||||||||||

Chapter 5

Coping Skills

We need to get one thing straight—something that not even many health gurus and diet specialists realize. As I mentioned before, you are not *under stress;* stress is inside you. *Pressure* is on the outside, and *stress* is on the inside. So you are *under pressure,* and this causes a *stress response,* which can be positive, negative, or neutral.

The human body loves positive stress responses. Achieving something good is a positive stress response, such as winning a race, getting a new job you've worked toward, or having a baby. There is no downside to that sort of stress. However, the human body does not enjoy negative stress responses piled one on top of the other. Eventually, this causes the body to break down and become unwell.

It's that pressure cooker I talked about in chapter 2. While you're in it, squirming under each additional bit of pressure, never forget that you have a choice in how you respond: you can react in a positive, neutral, or negative way. It's *always* your choice, even when you feel as if circumstances are working against you.

Though you may not appreciate the pressure you feel, you need to understand this: you cannot achieve anything of value without pressure, which can be external or applied by yourself. That means you need to learn to like pressure. If you want to get places and climb ladders—and we all do, frankly—you need to embrace pressure. In bursts, pressure can be quite stimulating. In big chronic lumps, however, it can be devastating.

Think about those little valves on the pressure cooker—the physical release valve (walking, stair climbing, etc.) and the psychological release valve (going to the beach, relaxing, etc.). These valves allow the whole thing to work. Take a minute to look back at the figure on page 49, which has lots of suggestions for releasing pressure.

When people start to stew, it's because they're staying in the pressure cooker 8 days a week, 57 weeks a year. This is where we get it wrong. The two valves are our means of escape (or at least of reducing pressure), and we need to use them liberally.

When you feel like you have to get out physically, open the physical release valve. What does that mean? As a short-term release, simply stretch. Or take a moment to just sit there and relax. Loosen your tie or blouse and take two or three deep breaths.

> Close your eyes for 60 seconds, think of someplace good, and take two or three gentle deep breaths, starting at the bottom of your lungs. I guarantee that you can lower your own blood pressure with this little trick—*and* you'll find yourself feeling far more relaxed.

The benefits of releasing pressure, or even jumping out of the pressure cooker for a time, are numerous. Among the most valuable:

- You start to see problems and hassles in a different light. With a new perspective may come a solution.
- You start to relax a bit, which lets you get excited about finding the *good* kind of stress response.

As a long-term approach, you have to commit 1 percent of your time to movement. As I previously mentioned, think of activity as another way to open the valve.

I have discussed with many people what they consider the best ways to get out of the pressure cooker and revitalize or reenergize their mind and their body. Everyone seems to have his or her own take on how best to relieve pressure. Take a walk. Wander around a botanical garden and smell the roses. Visit the zoo. Go to church. Listen to music.

Such a fabulous feeling—and you don't have to bust your gut doing it.

Laughter

Laughter is a great way to activate the pressure release valve. Lighten up a little. Stop taking everything so seriously—including yourself. Laugh at yourself. Go look in the mirror and make a face. If you're so serious that you can't laugh at that, then you're in serious trouble.

Laughter really is the best medicine. Laughter increases muscle tone in your neck, chest, and abdomen; and it can reduce your blood pressure as well as your levels of various stress hormones. Researchers have shown this to be fact.

Laughter may also build your immune system against cancerous activity, boosting your white blood cells—especially the kind known as T cells, which help combat tumor cells. Some types of white blood cells are sometimes referred to as "happy cells" because of their immune benefits.

Laughter also reduces the chance of respiratory infections, because laughing uses your full lung capacity. When you're stressed, you use only the top one-third of your lungs, which limits the amount of oxygen you're bringing into your system. When you laugh, however, you take deeper breaths. Utilizing your *entire* lungs helps clean out your system.

Laughter has been shown to increase memory and cognitive skills. People tend to remember conversations, lessons, and life advice better when humor is involved. I introduce (and practice) this whenever I speak at a convention, sit down for an interview, or run a group therapy session. One of my heroes is George Burns, because he had the ability to make other people laugh—and he laughed at himself—all the way to 100.

|||||||||||||||||||||||||||||||||||||||||||||||||||||||||||||||||||||||||||||||||||||

TICKELL TIP

Open your physical valve by skipping rope
3 or 5 or 10 or 20 times. Don't be afraid to play like
a kid. We too often tell kids to grow up, when
what we really need to do is grow down.

|||||||||||||||||||||||||||||||||||||||||||||||||||||||||||||||||||||||||||||||||||||

On top of everything else, laughter is contagious. Think, for a moment, about yawning. If you're in a room and three people are yawning, you start to yawn. If you're in a room and three people are laughing, you begin to laugh. So how can you make yourself laugh? Well, try going to a comedy show. Better yet, engage and mix with people who laugh easily. This brings into your life endless opportunities for laughter, which will help you—as it did George Burns—as you live and laugh your way to 100.

Laughter is medically positive. It's physically positive. And it's psychologically positive. No harm can ever come from laughing too much. Although you could die laughing, you'll never get sick laughing.

Bottom line, if you don't laugh, you're in trouble.

Seven-Minute Relaxation Session

People often tell me that they don't have time to relax. They're right. We're all busy, so in the interest of efficiency, let me share with you the shortest relaxation technique in the world. It's so short, all you need is seven minutes.

First, sit down and take off your shoes. Let the soles of your feet touch the floor so that you can feel the blood flow change.

Close your eyes, gently. Don't tense up your face. Just lightly close your eyes.

Concentrate on one sound. It could be a clock ticking. Or the hum of a fan or air conditioner. It could be music. My favorite sound to concentrate on is my own breathing. It's the easiest, I find; and the sound helps me link back up to the rhythm of my own body.

Take a couple of deep breaths through your diaphragm (the sheet of muscle between your chest and your stomach). Like a

[Blood Pressure]

You can't live without blood pressure. Blood pressure—it keeps you alive. If you've got no blood pressure, you're dead.

When the heart pumps, it pushes blood through the arteries at a particular pressure. That's the top measurement (the high point) of the blood pressure, and it's called the systolic blood pressure. That pressure, measured as the blood surges through, reflects the pressure when the heart is pumping, which it does somewhere between 50 and 100 times a minute.

(How often the heart beats is another story. If the heart is pumping fewer times per minute, it usually means it's fitter. And when your heart is fitter, it's more muscular and stronger and it can pump more blood per beat, which means it's more efficient. So if your heart is pumping more slowly to start with, when you expend energy and your heart rate fires up you can *produce* more energy and you get less tired. The fitter you are and the lower your resting heart rate, the more energy you have as the day goes on. It's a simple thing that many people don't understand: if you're sitting down and your heart is already banging away at 90 times a minute, you don't have much capacity to produce energy for long periods, so you become tired halfway through the afternoon.)

Now back to blood pressure. When the heart relaxes between beats, the pressure drops. It doesn't drop to nothing; it drops to what we call the diastolic level, which is a level lower than the systolic. Someone with training can actually hear these different sounds—pumping, resting—through the stethoscope. It's all to do with the ebb and flow of the blood going through the arteries because of the heart's pumping action.

Generally speaking, if you're considered low risk, the blood pressure should be less than, say, 140 for the top figure, and definitely less than 90 for the bottom one. And every tick or point above those levels gives you a higher risk associated with heart disease, heart attack, and stroke. Especially stroke.

So it's prudent to keep your blood pressure below 140 over 90. Of course, 130 over 85 is better, and 115 over 75 is sensational. The best way to reduce blood pressure is to have fewer blood vessels for the heart to pump the blood through. And given that every few pounds of fat require miles (true!) of additional blood vessels, why would you be overweight? Why add those miles and miles of extra pipes, putting the pressure up and making the pump work harder, which leads to higher blood pressure and a higher risk of stroke?

I repeat: take your heart for a walk around the block, climb stairs, forget the valet parking, and move at every opportunity. Get the weight off, lose those excess miles of blood vessels, tone up the 600 or so muscles in your body, and bring your blood pressure into the "healthy" zone. And let me tell you this. When you have achieved that transformation, you'll know all about it. You'll feel terrific!

singer, expand the bottom of your lungs, followed by the top. If you haven't been taught to breathe as a singer does, learn the Okinawan way: it's called abdominal breathing. As you slowly breathe in, hold the palm of one hand against your belly button and make sure it comes out two inches as you take a slow breath. As you breathe out, your belly button goes inward again! Two or three deep breaths from your diaphragm will help slow down your pulse and bring down your blood pressure.

When you're under pressure, you probably breathe with only the top third or half of your chest, quickly and inefficiently. You breathe 10 to 15 to 20 times a minute, typically. When the pressure's really on and you're either pumped or irritable, one of the two, you breathe in a more shallow fashion. The air is going up and down, yes, but you're not really getting much oxygen in your lungs because a lot of it is just moving up and down in the dead space of the windpipe. By breathing in with your diaphragm, however, you need only 4 or 6 breaths a minute instead of 10 or 20. This gives you a lot more oxygen per breath, as well as helping you relax and lowering your blood pressure.

Next, I want you to put your hands on your thighs and let your arms relax. Make sure the soles of your feet are flat on the floor. Breathe in and breathe out. Slow, deep breaths. You'll start to feel your pulse slow down, perhaps in your chest or the side of your head.

Take another breath, slowly and deeply, again from the diaphragm.

Start to contract your left leg. Tighten your thigh and calf muscles, then claw up your foot as hard as you can. Hold for five seconds, then let it go and relax. Take another breath, slowly and deeply, again from the diaphragm.

In normal circumstances, you can feel an increase in temperature, an increase in warmth in the sole of your foot, as the blood vessels open out. Your leg feels heavy and relaxed.

Take another breath, slowly and deeply, again from the diaphragm.

Now contract your right leg. Tighten your thigh and calf muscles, then claw up your foot as hard as you can. Hold for five seconds, then let it go and relax. Feel the warmth in the sole of your foot.

Take another breath, slowly and deeply, again from the diaphragm.

Below the waist, your limbs are heavy and very relaxed.

Now contract your left arm. Squeeze it into your body, contracting your biceps. Draw your forearm up to your chest and clench your fist as hard as you can. Hold for five seconds, then let it go and relax. Your fingers should warm from the increased blood flow.

Take another breath, slowly and deeply, again from the diaphragm.

Now contract your right arm. Squeeze it into your body, contracting your biceps. Draw your forearm up to your chest and clench your fist as hard as you can. Hold for five seconds, then let it go and relax. Your fingers should warm from the increased blood flow.

Like your legs, your arms should now feel heavy and relaxed.

Now the stomach. Pull your belly button back toward your spine and squeeze your stomach up. Hold for five seconds, then let it go and relax.

Take another breath, slowly and deeply, again from the diaphragm.

||||||||||||||||||||||||||||||||||||||||||||||||||||||||||||||||||||||||||||||||||||

TICKELL TIP

Whenever you see some paper or rubbish
on the floor, pick it up and put it in the trash. Picking up
things from the floor helps keep you flexible.
Bend your knees, not your back.

||||||||||||||||||||||||||||||||||||||||||||||||||||||||||||||||||||||||||||||||||||

Now the neck. Bring your chin(s) up toward your teeth. Chins up. Hold for five seconds, then let it go and relax.

Take another breath, slowly and deeply, again from the diaphragm.

Your neck should feel heavy and relaxed.

Last one. We'll do the eyes and the scalp together. Bring your hairline (wherever it might be) down to your eyebrows and scrunch up your eyes. Tighten them as hard as you can. You'll start to see different colors and shapes: blue and black, circles and squiggles. Hold for five seconds, then let them go and relax.

Take another breath, slowly and deeply, again from the diaphragm.

Your eyes and scalp should feel heavy and relaxed.

This whole process usually takes three or four minutes. Take the next three or four minutes to daydream. Let your mind wander to a beach or a grove of orange trees or a windswept plain or a snow-capped mountain. It's your choice. As you go there, continue to breathe easily, in and out, slowly, from the diaphragm.

While relaxation is important, so is activity. Take the time to walk around the office for 30 or 60 seconds once every hour. Wave and say hello to your colleagues. If people frown at you, pull a face and grin at them. But do walk hourly. If there are stairs in your office, make sure to go up or down them (or both) during your trip around the office. That takes a little more time, but it also produces a little more benefit.

Mental Bonuses

Mental bonuses are things that you look forward to but rarely get around to doing. Things you should be doing, for your health and well-being, but hardly ever do.

Type A maniacs never buy a book; they don't buy a racy novel and read a chapter now and then. They don't go to movies. They don't lie on beaches. They don't fish. They never walk around a garden on a lazy Sunday and smell the roses. They don't think they have the time or patience to do such things.

But you do have the time. This is the B-time I wrote about in chapter 2. The out-of-the-pressure-cooker time. If you don't get out of the pressure cooker, you'll stew yourself. You'll break down, eventually—hopefully with just a migraine and not a heart scare.

The greatest mental bonus ever invented is the three-day, three-times-a-year switch-off. Just three days once every four months. That's a total of nine days out of several hundred *just for you*. It might seem a bit selfish, but I'll tell you what: it works.

No work. No home. You have to get away—anywhere. Block off three days in your date book or diary four months out. The human brain loves looking forward to things, and every time you're hassled, at least you'll have something out there to think about.

I can feel you tensing up right now. There's always something to do, especially if you're a type A person. But this works wonders even for you maniacs. Getting away three times a year actually gives you a chance to get *more* things done. You can get really clever a couple of weeks before your break. You might start to delegate more in anticipation. With five days left, you might work late or come in early to finish up a few last things. You just sweep

[Worry]

The majority of people react to pressure by engaging in what I call corridor thinking. That's when you think up and down in an enclosed space and use only about 15 percent of your brainpower. This is conservative thinking. It's not very adventurous; it's safe.

It's not a bad idea to start thinking sideways sooner rather than later, because things might start to get even worse, and if the walls of your mental corridor start to close in, you'll need a contingency plan, a way out. Sideways thinking is also known as lateral thinking. It's just another way of looking at things.

As soon as children think of something, they say it. Kids are brilliant at lateral thinking because it's so natural for them. Adults laugh at things kids say because we think they're funny, but kids don't think they're funny. They think their approach is perfectly normal.

That's because kids' brains haven't been squeezed shut by society, by the social and corporate rules that tell us, "Do this, not that." Kids' minds are free, unburdened by the chains of conformity. They think upward, downward, sideways, and every which way.

Unfortunately, as kids grow up, they lose this trait, just as we did, especially when the pressure is on.

I want you to try something. Draw a straight line down the middle of a blank page of paper. On one side, write "Can Do." On

it all away and off you go. And, once you return, you'll discover that the world hasn't fallen apart.

There are, by my count, three different types of breaks.

The first is the selfish break, when you do the getaway on your

the other, write "Can't Do." These two columns represent what you can and can't do about the things you're worried about. List all the things you're currently worried about in the appropriate column. Are you worried about taxes? Your mother-in-law? Well, I'm sorry, but you can't do anything about either of those things. Put them in the Can't Do column. You'll soon realize that you can forget about most of your worries, since you can't fix them anyway. You'll just have to coexist peaceably with them.

One of the great things about the brain is all of its wonderful compartments. You can put a worry that you can't do anything about into one of those little boxes in the side of your brain and lock it up and forget about it.

Set aside 20 minutes a day to write down everything you're worried about that you can't do anything about and then store that entire list—the entire Can't Do column—in one of those neat little mental boxes.

What about the Can Dos? Well, *do* something about them. Create a management plan. Take action. Then cross them off your list because they've been taken care of.

Why waste so much of your life worrying about things you can't do anything about, while refusing to deal with the worrisome things you can do something about? Life is for the living.

own. The second is the spouse or partner break: you and your significant other get away from work, kids, and the daily routine for those three days. This is an important kind of break. Relationships are a work in progress, which means you have to work at them. I've been with my wonderful wife for more than 40 years and we have five kids. She and I always sneak away three or four times a year.

TICKELL TIP

Take your partner away for three days, three times
a year. While you're away, have a cocktail and watch a
sunset together, or go to the beach or mountains.

The third type of break is the family vacation, which often causes more stress in people. But, as with everything else in life, it all comes down to your attitude. Keep things simple, make sure there's something of interest for everyone, and relax!

The Horizon

There's a line, like the horizon, that I call the Thinking Line.

When your business hits a bump or your cat dies, you start to worry or grieve and you get a little down. Your spirit sinks. Your attitude sours. And you dive under the line.

How long do you want to stay there when things go bad? An hour? A week? Three months? Most winners come up again relatively quickly. They spend 80 percent of their time thinking above the line.

How you choose to think is how you do think. Your mind is your greatest asset. It will let you down only if you allow it to let you down. Keep those ridiculous worries locked up in those little boxes, where you can take them out every now and then examine them at your discretion.

Sleep

Sleep is magic stuff. It happens when the bacterial and other debris builds up in your body and your system needs to rejuvenate itself.

We spend up to one-third of our life sleeping. Don't think of this as wasted time, though; it can be very useful. Large chunks of our life are spent standing in lines and worrying about things we can do nothing about. Now *that* is relatively useless.

Are America's 20 to 40 million insomniacs at a disadvantage? Possibly, but people who "can't sleep" actually sleep more than they think they do—and besides, some of us get more sleep than we need.

You can't die from not sleeping, just like you can't die by holding your breath. If you're holding your breath, eventually you will faint and breathe again; and even if you're the world's worst insomniac, eventually you will fall asleep.

The average human being needs between 6 and 8 hours of sleep every 24 hours to maintain an effective immune system, keep the emotions on a relatively even keel, be physically well and mentally sharp, and have reflex and coordination performances in top shape.

Did you know that poor sleeping habits can be tied up with being overweight? Well, many scientists say that they can.

Too little sleep can cause you to become a real mess, as can too *much* sleep. So how do you get a good night's sleep?

Here are some tricks:

- Physically tired people sleep better than mentally tired people. *Fact.* If you walk through the hills with a pack on your back, you'll sleep *well* that night!
- Try a relaxation technique. Slow breathing is the beginning point. Buy a book and read all about it.
- Do some numbers in your head. Count backward. Keep subtracting by 7s from 300 until you get near 0. (If you do get to 0, you're wrong—start again!)
- Close your eyes and think about wonderful things. Fantasize a little—maybe a beach and a palm tree.
- Have a treat. Maybe a nice glass of wine to settle you down—but one glass only!

Sunshine

Sunshine is similarly good for your body—and especially good for your mind. A decent burst of sunshine makes you feel good; sunlight elevates the mood and does good things with vitamin D and calcium metabolism. There are heaps of people in the world who are vitamin D–deficient because they choose to hide from the sun.

Still, you do have to be careful not to get too much sun, especially if you have fair skin. No sun-baking between 10:00 A.M. and 2:00 P.M., when the rays are at their strongest. Although I don't think you need to run away from the sunshine, you should *not* burn your skin in the hot sun. Remember, moderation in every-thing. If you're concerned about spots and moles and things changing shape or color, visit your skin specialist. *Now.*

I have a friend who is a good dermatologist—he started from scratch! (Sorry: couldn't resist.)

If everyone had a peaches-and-cream complexion, it would be boring, wouldn't it? I like a few wrinkles here and there, if only to make people think I'm wise.

Vitamins

Vitamins and other micronutrients are substances that make the biochemical magic of our bodies possible—producing energy and making body tissues, blood cells, and hormones.

These nutrients, found primarily in plant-based foods, are also necessary to maintain the immune system in tip-top shape, increas-ing resistance against infections and cancers.

Stressful living and polluted air use up large quantities of the vitamins in our bodies, which is why it's so important that people who live and work in pressure-cooker environments eat very, very well. Unfortunately, usually they do just the opposite: the more pressure people are under, the more junk they typically eat.

There is some evidence to suggest that the taking of nutritional supplements can pump up the immune system and increase resis-tance to various diseases, including cancers. The antioxidant group (more on this later) can scavenge excess "free" radicals, the nasty by-products of a metabolism under pressure. Millions and millions of free radicals are produced by a body that eats lousy food, is slobbishly inactive, worries too much, smokes, and drinks lots of booze—in short, a body that is coping poorly with the pressures of life.

Excess free radicals are also produced by bodies that exercise to excess, are very intense, and maybe don't sleep so well. Being aggressive and unfriendly doesn't help either.

The human system needs a few free radicals, but if you have too many wandering around inside you, they stuff up your immune system and you can become more prone to colds, flu, cancers, and illness in general. Apart from that, you age faster than the calendar. Understand? You get older quicker.

I'm convinced that all the various micronutrients act in concert, like an orchestra. If only the tuba player and the violinist show up, the music doesn't sound so good, but if the whole orchestra is there, you hear a great performance—especially if the conductor is there as well.

So eat your vegetables, fruits, grains, nuts, and seeds—the wider the variety, the better it is for you. And the more different colors of plant foods, the better your body responds. Plant foods definitely have more healthy micronutrients than flesh foods—just look at the evidence: the longest-living, healthiest people on the planet.

Everyday Relaxation List

I have discussed with many successful people the best ways they know to get out of the pressure cooker. What follows is a suggested Relaxation List (by no means complete). Choose several items from the list (or add your own) and place them in your life regularly. To score your Living*life* points, you need to do one or two each day.

Relaxation List

- Go to one of these destinations—a mountain, forest, beach, stream, or pool; sit there, walk there, or lie there
- Watch a sunrise
- Watch a sunset
- Go to a movie
- Have coffee with a friend
- Sit in the sunshine
- Lie in the sunshine
- Sip a glass of really good wine
- Read a book
- Swim in the ocean
- Have a warm bath
- Light a candle
- Listen to relaxing music
- Do some deep breathing
- Get a massage
- Get a facial
- Plan your next three-day break
- Have a cup of tea and do a crossword puzzle
- Close your eyes and dream of good things
- Call someone you haven't seen for a while
- Go to an old-folks home and have a chat
- Practice tai chi

When you have a problem, there may be more than one way to tackle it—and tackling it will help you relax. Think of alternative approaches when you face an obstacle, and if things are not clear, involve somebody else and seek his or her advice. Women are habitually better at seeking advice than men. Surprise!

Positive reinforcement on a regular basis is excellent. Encouragement helps you feel good about yourself and relax. Be sure to *offer* encouragement to others as well!

Check out your behavior type—A, B, C, or maybe AB. Work on it if you need to. Be aware of your responses to people and events.

Monitor your aggression level and how things build up inside you—and how long it takes you to calm down.

Think good things and dream a little.

Put time into your relationships. Do you have your next three-day partner break planned yet? If not, call a travel agent or look online and get some brochures. Do you ever wonder why 30 to 50 percent of marriages break down? Don't be among that group!

Did you get your laugh, hug, relaxation, sleep, and good-person points today?

If yes—sensational. If no—why not?

Why is that so important? Because if you're doing the things we're talking about here, you'll feel ever so much better about yourself and about life.

Today's Coping List	
Every day you need to ask yourself these questions:	
Good sleep last night?	Yes
Deep breathing?	Yes
Laugh?	Yes
Hug?	Yes
Something good for someone else?	Yes
Another item from the Relaxation List?	Yes

||||||||||||||||||||||||||||||||||||||||||||||||||||||||||||||||||||||

TICKELL TIP

You control 80 percent of *everything*

that happens to you. This is a simple fact of life.

Most of us, however, lack self-responsibility.

We immediately start blaming everyone

else for whatever goes wrong.

Take responsibility!

||||||||||||||||||||||||||||||||||||||||||||||||||||||||||||||||||||||

Attitude Adjustment

Without doubt, "attitude" is the most important word in the English language. And the sad fact of life is that more and more people today look at the downside rather than the upside. The weather forecast is "partly cloudy" rather than "partly sunny."

We wake to a new day, and instead of celebrating the fact that we're alive and can do good things today, we worry about what's going to go wrong. Tornados, hurricanes, terrorism, plane crashes, mortgage foreclosures, businesses going bankrupt. Everything in the headlines is negative, so we need to be strong in order to look at the bright side of life, at the positive things. One of the greatest problems we have in our life is news media. Negative headlines sell.

Another major problem is social media. A psychologist recently discovered that nearly 50 percent of comments on social media are negative. That's huge!

We don't control our lives; our lives control us—or at least that's how it feels most of the time. We need to reflect on who or what is controlling which parts of our lives. Is television dictating what we think? The stock market? Online bullying? Our taste buds? Fear?

So what are we going to do about this? As with most things in life, it all comes back to looking in the mirror. We are self-responsible for what goes on in our lives. What we need is a change of attitude, and we need to keep it simple: we don't want to be confused while we're changing our attitude.

Breaking the cycle is not difficult. It's simply a matter of choosing to live a better, more positive life.

|||||||||||||||||||||||||||||||||||||||||||||||||||||||||||||||||||||||||||||||||||||||||||||||||||||

Chapter 6

Eating Skills

Don't listen to what everyone else tells you about not eating this and doubling your intake of that. Eating is easy: all you have to do is . . . the right thing! Get smart and follow the guidelines, because your "machine" is depending on you.

As I wrote in chapter 3, the human machine can live a long and healthy life on Basic Foods alone—that is, plant foods (vegetables, fruits, grains, nuts, and seeds)—with the occasional touch of animal flesh or other Bonus Foods every now and again. The human machine cannot, however, live a long and healthy life on flesh and other Bonus Foods alone—although one could be forgiven for thinking that. Plenty of high-protein diet experts have written books proclaiming this, after all.

Plant foods—Basic Foods—contain thousands of different micronutrients that make the human machine run superbly. We know from the longest-living and healthiest people on earth—our friends,

[The Top 10 Favorite Foods
of the Longest-Living People on Earth]

Rice

Fish

Soybeans

Goya (the closest Western equivalent is zucchini)

Sweet potatoes

Firm tofu

Miso paste and miso soup

Seaweed

Shiitake mushrooms

Jasmine tea

the Okinawans—that the best endorphin-producing foods are plant foods. Certain Basic Foods, including broccoli and blueberries, have incredibly many micronutrients in them, particularly antioxidants. (More on those so-called superfoods in the next chapter.)

People say, "What's an antioxidant, Doctor?" To answer that question, let's start with a close relative of that word, "oxidation," which is the process of aging—in effect, of rusting. When you cut an apple in two halves and leave the flesh exposed to the air, what color does it turn? Brown. It rusts! That's called oxidation. The same thing happens to you as you age—you *rust*. And that makes you get older quicker.

*Anti*oxidants, chemicals that counter the oxidization process, are found in natural foods—that is, foods that haven't been processed or refined. Foods like spinach and broccoli and berries. Scientists tell us that blueberries have more antioxidants than any other food on earth. Antioxidants are packed with cancer-fighting phytochemicals (more on these in the next chapter too) that help slow down the aging process. They hold off the rusting, as it were. It's no accident, then, that the longest-living people in the world live on antioxidant-rich Basic Foods, while we Westerners only occasionally order such foods as sides.

Bonus Foods, on the other hand, contain far fewer nutrients. They also have a ton of additives. Humans have a nasty habit of messing around with food. This never used to be the case. Unfortunately, it's now the norm. And it's not good, not good at all.

You could draw a line down the middle of a page and list the ways that Bonus Foods are tampered with in two categories: "Before Picked or Killed" and "After Picked or Killed." The obvi-

As we saw in an earlier chapter, there are good oils and not-so-good oils. Good oils include extra-virgin olive oil and flaxseed oil, although you can't cook in flaxseed oil. I give them an HI of zero. They're made up of healthy and stable saturated and monounsaturated fats, which are essential for the absorption of most nutrients. The longest-living (documented and verified) person on the planet was Jeanne Calment of France, who lived to be 122 years and 164 days. Her secret of living life? "Everything I ate," she said, "I added olive oil." She also rubbed it on her skin.

Not-so-good oils include canola, sunflower, corn, and safflower oils, which are often labeled, generically, as vegetable oil. I give these an HI of 1. (For more information about good and bad oils, see the appendix, page 217.)

ous Befores include things like antibiotics, steroids, hormones, and pesticides—among hundreds, if not thousands, of other chemicals. The Afters include chemical additives, preservatives, dyes, salt, sugar, and artificial flavoring—not to mention preparation methods such as microwave radiation and deep-frying.

Human interference—measured by the HI index I mentioned in an earlier chapter—has transformed many of our foods from natural to not-so-natural.

Do you think Okinawans go to supermarkets? Of course not. They go to *real* markets. They don't need to read labels or try to divine what's in their food from a cryptic list of ingredients, includ-

---

I don't want to tell you what to eat. You can eat whatever you want. I just want you to *think* about what you're eating. I want you to wonder why you need a huge muffin instead of only a couple of bites. Why you need three doughnuts instead of one or none. Why you need two scoops of ice cream instead of one (or some sorbet) on your fresh fruit. Are you feeding your stomach and head, or are you just feeding your tongue?

To make sure you're taking care of your head and your stomach, start grazing—in other words, eating small bits of many things, several times a day. This is a great way to moderate and level out blood glucose, which (when kept at a good level) sustains our thinking power and good energy throughout the day.

The American lifestyle seems to revolve around two or three larger meals, but when we go back to those clever people who live into their 90s and 100s with good brainpower, we discover that they tend to graze on foods; they're eating a little, but often. Now, you might say, "Well, that's impossible, Doctor, because I go

ing hard-to-read chemical formulas and artificial dye numbers. Vegetables and fruits and fish don't need labels.

We need to get away from food with a high HI rating, especially anything that's processed or deep-fried. We need to start eating food with a low HI rating—the lower the better.

As I wrote earlier, this isn't rocket science. You don't need to count grams or ounces or carbs or calories, nor do you need to step on scales every day. This isn't about losing weight. It's about winning. And how do winners in life come out on top? They use their brains. Which means all you have to do is think. And once you start to think, you'll start to win.

---

out to lunch to get away from the office, so I have a big meal and a glass of wine to help me relax. Then I go home after work and my partner and I make a big dinner and I pour another glass of wine. I eat and drink it all up and then I go to bed."

Think about it, though: When you go to bed, what do you do with all the calories? You burn only 50 or 60 calories an hour when you're asleep. When you're awake and sitting at your desk, you're burning 90 to 100 calories an hour, which may not be great but is at least better. So why would you eat all that food at the end of the day? The best way to level out your blood glucose is by minding the old adage, "Breakfast like a king, lunch like a prince, and dine like a pauper." It's the exact opposite of the way we tend to do things: we don't eat breakfast at all, we have some lunch (a sandwich and maybe a little something on the side—a muffin, say, and a coffee), and then at nighttime we take in a huge number of calories.

Think and Win

This is so easy that you'll get the hang of it quickly. I'll start you off with general guidelines, along with specific examples. In no time, you'll be able to work out the HI index of every type of food, whether Basic or Bonus.

We do need to give nature some credit here for creating decent, wholesome food. That means we start with an HI rating of zero, indicating a real whole food.

From zero, I start adding up. I mentally go through a list of what might have happened to a food before it was picked or killed, and I add an HI point for every not-so-real thing. I then work out what happened to the food after it was harvested. Finally, I decide whether or not I'm going to eat it (and if yes, how much of it I'm going to eat—all of it or just a little).

I do this for everything I eat, with one major exception: anything deep-fried. I don't add a single point for frying; I *double* however many points there are. In other words, if something has an HI rating of 4 before cooking, I give it an 8 if it's deep-fried. That's how frighteningly bad deep-fried food is for you. The level of human interference in fried food is twice as high as that of the underlying food, which may already be pretty bad for you.

That's it. Pretty simple, right? Look at foods individually and then look at the whole meal. Then ask yourself if it fulfills the Four Simple Rules of Nutrition that were introduced in chapter 3. Let's review those rules here:

Rule 1: Basic and Bonus

Think about whether the foods are Basic or Bonus.

Easy—plant or not plant.

Rule 2: Two-Thirds, One-Third

Does *at least* two-thirds of the meal consist of Basic Foods? Easy. Consider a meal made up of fish and salad or vegetables plus some fries. The salad and vegetables are Basic Foods; the fish is Bonus Food, but a great Bonus because of its omega-3 content and low HI. The fries are technically from a plant, but let's not get carried away. Think about what humans have done to the potato to turn it into fries—clearly a high HI. So I'll eat just 6 fries instead of 30 or 300.

Rule 3: HI Instead of GI

Does my meal rate low on the HI index? Absolutely. The fries have been totally wrecked by HI, but since I'm eating just a few, they don't torpedo the meal.

Rule 4: The Rule of 15

Is this meal helping me toward my 15 plant foods for the day? Yes.

The only tough decision is, Can I walk away from 294 fries?

I can. I just visualize what they would do to the inside of my human machine. It's not worth the risk.

||||||||||||||||||||||||||||||||||||||||||||||||||||||||||||||||||||||||||||||||||

TICKELL TIP

The most important weight-loss organ in your body is located between your ears. When people go on a diet, their thinking is usually in the wrong space; it's best to think with your brain, not your tongue or your stomach. Keep your brain happy by keeping your taste buds and your stomach happy.

||||||||||||||||||||||||||||||||||||||||||||||||||||||||||||||||||||||||||||||||||

The HI List

Preharvest Interference

To determine a food's HI index, add 1 point for each of the following *pre*harvest forms of interference:

- Chemical enhancements like steroids, antibiotics, fertilizers, pesticides
- Artificial growth factors like light, heat, unnatural feed
- Genetic modification (GM)

Postharvest Interference

Now adjust the HI index by adding 1 point for each of the following *post*harvest forms of interference:

- Refining
- Processing
- Artificial preserving
- Coloring
- Using additives
- Making subtractions
- Packaging
- Storing long-term
- Peeling, slicing, dicing, mashing, smashing, pureeing
- Salting (pepper is okay)
- Sugaring
- Oiling
- Overcooking
- Saucing

Exceptions

Packaging
- Don't add HI 1 for frozen food. HI 0 is fine.
- Some basic foods in a box or can are fine—for example, whole-grain cereals and canned vegetable soups.

Oiling

- Don't add HI 1 for a little added olive oil, flaxseed oil, or soybean oil; HI 0 is fine for small amounts.
- If oils are solid, like canola in a tub, add HI 1.

Cooking

- Don't add HI 1 for lightly steaming food, lightly cooking food in a wok, or quickly dropping food into boiling water; HI 0 is fine by me. As for microwaving, I don't add HI 1 for a microwave zap—I stick with HI 0—but you might; it's your call.
- My cooking HI ratings go like this:

Lightly steaming	0
Lightly cooking in wok	0
Quickly dropping into boiling water	0
Microwaving	0–1
Grilling	1
Boiling	1
Baking	1
Roasting	1
Smoking	1
Barbecuing	2
Deep-frying	*Double the HI index!*

Fluids

- Water is HI 0.
- Green tea and black tea are HI 0.
- Don't add HI 1 for up to two cups of coffee per day.
- Don't add HI 1 for the following:
    Sips of skim milk
    Any amount of non-GM soy milk

Sauces/Dressings

- Add HI 1 for any sauce or dressing except (a little) olive oil and vinegar.

After a while, you'll be able to assess a food in a few seconds. It's either good or fair or a total health disaster. Calculating the *precise* HI index isn't all that important.

Here are some real-life examples.

Example 1: An Apple

Might have been sprayed, which means it needs to be washed. It most likely ripened naturally, in the sunshine.

At this stage, the apple's index is around HI 1.

Going along the good to not-so-good scale, the progression continues.

> Apple picked, washed, and eaten whole—still HI 0
>
> Apple put in Grandma's apple pie (with big chunks of apple and a little pastry): apple peeled and stewed (add HI 1); sugar added (add HI 1); pastry made with refined flour (add HI 1)—HI 3
>
> Apple in store-bought apple muffin with a few bits of cooked apple (add HI 1), along with huge amounts of sugar (1), refined flour (1), and trans fat (1)—HI 4 or more
>
> Apple in fast-food apple pie: peeled, smashed, sugared, and prepared with refined flour (HI 4); that number doubled if it's fried—HI 8!

Example 2: A Potato

> Let's pretend it grew up without interference—HI 0
>
> What did I do to it? I peeled, sliced, diced, and mashed it—HI 1
>
> What did I add to it? Salt and butter—HI 2

How did I cook it? I baked it with olive oil—HI 1

Total—HI 4

If I were rating french fries, the HI would be doubled because of the deep-frying, so I'd give them an HI of at least 6. Wouldn't you agree?

And don't forget that it's a *quantity* thing as well. There's a difference between a couple of small, real potatoes and a veritable truckload of fries.

Remember, we're not trying to get too technical here. This isn't an exam. It's a great way of working out, in general terms, how junky or useless a particular food is. Or, on the other hand, how real it is.

Most important, you must begin to recognize the factors that give foods a high HI rating and start to avoid them.

Example 3: Chicken

Here are some chicken ideas for you . . .

How was it raised? Probably under lights—HI 1

What did it eat? Most likely unnatural pellets—HI 1

It was probably given a host of other elements, such as steroids and antibiotics—HI 2

What happened to it? It was killed, plucked, and packed in plastic or foam—HI 1

What part of it am I eating?
- Breast—HI 0
- Legs and skin—HI 1 for each

The reason for the different scoring is that the breast is usually prepared in chunks and cooked without the skin, which means that no fat has seeped into it from the skin during cooking; legs, on the other hand, are skinny, so fat seeps in easily from the skin. (Chicken skin is *very fatty*.)

How was it cooked?
- Boiled—HI 1
- Grilled—HI 1
- Deep-fried—multiply final HI by 2

Has it been reheated? HI 1

Let's say we're eating a reheated skin-on chicken leg that was deep-fried; we bought it, wrapped in foam and plastic, from a supermarket; and the bird from which the meat came originally was force-fed pellets under lights and given steroids to make it grow faster. I'd give that chicken leg about a 13!

In fact, it should have had flashing red lights all around it in the store's display.

Are you getting the picture? Whether you think that the chicken leg's HI rating should be 10, 12, 14, or 200 doesn't really matter. What matters is that this reheated chicken is a disaster.

And don't forget that eating reheated chicken is a good way to give yourself the upset-tummy syndrome (or food poisoning).

Example 4: Fish

What sort of fish?
- Deep-sea, cold-water fish—HI 0
- Farm-grown fish—HI 2
- Bottom-dwelling crustacean—HI 1

How did it arrive?

- Straight from market—HI 0
- In a can—HI 0–1 (it's your decision)

How was it cooked?

- Wok with canola oil or lightly steamed—HI 0
- Wok with saturated fat oil—HI 1
- Grilled or baked—HI 0–1 (it's your decision)
- Deep-fried—multiply final HI by 2

Was anything added?

- Salt—HI 1
- Sauce—HI 1
- Lemon—HI 0

Let's say the fish we prepared was a deep-sea fish (salmon) that came straight from the market, and it was cooked in a wok with canola oil and served with some added lemon, chives, or parsley.

Hey, the index is close to HI 0. You beauty! Add a few vegetables and you're really rocking and rolling.

Get the picture?

I told you it was easy. And it's fun.

It's your call now, because you have all the basic information at your fingertips.

As I said—all you need to do is *think and win.*

PART THREE

Love, Laugh, and Eat and Beyond

||||||||||||||||||||||||||||||||||||||||||||||||||||||||||||||||||||||||||||||||||||||||||||||||||||||||||||||||||||||||||

Chapter 7

Superfoods

Is there such a thing as a superfood? Browsing through magazines, one often comes across advertisements for products touted as such—extracts of something or other that could be "the answer to life."

My reading of the situation is this: yes, there are superfoods; and no, there isn't one particular superfood. While superfoods let you absorb more nutrients with less eating, there is, as yet, no magic bullet. Nor, I'm quite sure, will there ever be.

If you eat right across the range of superfoods, however, you're in business. As powerful sources of protein, vitamins, minerals, enzymes, antioxidants, and other nutrients, the aptly named superfoods can offer extraordinary dietary and health benefits.

The best kinds of superfoods are "green"; that is, they're plant-based foods—the Basic Foods we talked about in chapter 3. These

vegetables, fruits, grains, nuts, and seeds contain a high concentration of nutrients, including vitamins, minerals, and clean proteins that help keep you lean, clean, and free from disease. All
green vegetables are full of antioxidants—and the darker the
green, the better. Other carcinogen blockers (known as pungent
preventives) come in allium vegetables, such as garlic and onions.
Garlic has long been considered an immune system booster—
something to do with the sulfur compounds.

Rather than focusing on a specific superfood, I'd like to high-
light the many benefits of the superfood family—that is, Basic
Foods. Let's look at what's in those foods that makes them super.

Antioxidants

Of course, the big rage these days is antioxidants, and with good
reason. It seems that certain foods, or what's in them, can potentially block the chemicals that can initiate the cancer process. Let
me tell you this: a person's cancer did not start last week or last
month, out of the blue. Most people develop rapidly dividing cells
(mitotic cells), or precancerous cells, quite commonly. It's up to
your immune system to knock these out. If your immune system
isn't strong enough to wipe out these cells, they may be the start
of a cancerous growth or tumor.

In chapter 5 I introduced the concept of free radicals, which
are a by-product of metabolism, and which (though necessary in
small numbers) can damage your immune system. Antioxidants
can snuff out excess free radicals—the nasties, as I like to call
them—and may even repair cellular damage. Some of the most
effective antioxidants are vitamin C (found in citrus fruits, straw-

---

[Probiotics]

Not all bacteria are bad. Some are good for you. Probiotics are beneficial bacteria that inhabit the human gut. You may be surprised to hear that there are 4 to 10 times as many probiotic cells in your intestines as there are cells in the rest of your body! Probiotics help you break down and digest your food, and they protect you from organisms that cause disease. An unhealthy diet or an overreliance on antibiotics can kill good bacteria, which will mess up your digestion and can rob you of valuable nutrients.

One of the best ways to flood your body with probiotics—and push out unhealthy bacteria—is through fermented and cultured foods such as yogurt, kimchi, sauerkraut, raw apple-cider vinegar, kombucha tea, pickles, and kefir.

---

berries, and potatoes), vitamin E (nuts, grains, certain oils, and leafy greens), and beta-carotene (carrots, apricots, peaches, cantaloupes, sweet potatoes, and spinach). It is truly amazing that ordinary fruits and vegetables can be so effective against carcinogens.

Beta-Carotene

The precursor of vitamin A or, if you like, the plant form of vitamin A, beta-carotene is high on the antioxidant list of superfoods. It is found in yellow, orange, and deep-green foods such as carrots, apricots, peaches, cantaloupes, sweet potatoes, and spinach.

Phytochemicals

Phytochemicals—literally, plant chemicals—are naturally occurring compounds, many of which are suspected or known to have health benefits for humans. They stack up particularly well in cruciferous vegetables, soybeans, onions, and citrus fruit. Cruciferous vegetables, as you may know, hail from the cabbage family. They include cabbage, cauliflower, brussels sprouts, broccoli, kale, and bok choy. "Cruciferous" comes from the word "crucifix"—the leaves and petals cross each other.

Many people say to me, "I just don't like them." I say, "Well, *get* to like them! That's where all the micronutrient action is."

Research suggests that if you eat foods rich in phytochemicals day after day, it's more difficult for breast cancer, colon cancer, and other cancers to take hold in your body. But don't overcook these foods or you might destroy the indoles—whatever they are. (They're possibly the cancer crunchers.)

Lycopene

Lycopene, a bright red carotene, can help prevent certain types of cancer, according to scientific research. Tomatoes, for instance—rich in lycopene—may offer good protection against prostate cancer, which is why every male in the world should eat a tomato or tomato product every day. (Ironically, cooked tomato is better than raw for this purpose.) Lycopene is also found in red bell peppers, apricots, watermelons, and some other red fruits and vegetables.

[Soya, Tofu, and Miso]

Around 3,000 years ago, the Chinese discovered a wild berry they called the *soya*. As they domesticated the plant, it began to produce larger seeds, which became their source of bean sprouts, milk, sauces, flour, and cooking oil.

Tofu is a soya bean (or, more typically now, *soybean*) product, made by grinding, boiling, and draining soybeans and curdling their milk to form a solid but workable substance. Long since having spread worldwide from China, this substance is now offered as a primary ingredient to make cheesecake, lasagna, quiche, moussaka, and many other foods.

Also growing in popularity are tofu and soy milk–based nondairy frozen desserts.

Science tells us that there is a positive connection between the consumption of soy foods and the reduction of the risk of heart disease and hardening of the arteries. The substitution of vegetable protein (from soybeans) for much of our animal protein is a definite positive for the heart, and it's fabulous for diabetes as well.

Firm Tofu

Dense and solid, firm tofu holds up well in stir-fry dishes, in soups, and on the grill. Firm tofu is also higher in protein and calcium than any other form of tofu.

Soft Tofu

Soft tofu is great for recipes that call for blended tofu and in Asian soups.

(continued . . .)

Silken Tofu

A creamy, custard-like product, silken tofu works well in pureed or blended dishes. In Japan, silken tofu is enjoyed "as is," with just a touch of soy sauce and chopped spring onions.

Miso

A rich and savory paste made from fermented soybeans and a yeast-like mold—which can come from rice, barley, or soy— miso is one of Japan's most important foods. It is rich in amino acids, vitamins, and minerals, and packed with active enzymes. It is most famously used in miso soup, but it's also used as an instant seasoning for dips, salads, marinades, and other soups.

Flavonoids

Flavonoids are plant compounds found in soy products, flaxseed, onions, cranberries, grapes, apples, broccoli, and some teas, including jasmine tea. A group of plant substances with recognized antioxidant properties, flavonoids help fight inflammation. Dried and canned beans—chickpeas, lentils, kidney beans, pinto beans, navy beans, black beans, pink beans, and white beans—are also on the good guys' list.

It's worth noting that the risk of developing hormone-dependent cancers in countries that consume high quantities of soy products and other flavonoid-containing foods is dramatically lower than in Western countries. Soybeans and soy products seem to play a part in the cancer prevention business, especially colon, breast, and prostate cancers. Soy products include natural soybeans, tofu, miso paste and soup, soy milk, soy flour, and roasted soybeans (soy nuts). Soybeans also contain phytoestrogen, or plant estrogen.

Soluble and Insoluble Fiber

Soluble and insoluble fiber in various foods have been shown in several studies to lower cholesterol levels (soluble fiber) and potentially help reduce the risk of colon cancer (insoluble fiber).

Soluble fiber is found in fruit, rice, and oat bran. Insoluble fiber is found in rinds, whole grains, corn, and many other vegetables.

[Whole Grains and Rice]

In addition to providing valuable vitamins and minerals, whole grains have protective powers. Studies have shown that people who regularly consume quantities of whole grains are much less likely to develop type 2 diabetes. Because whole grains slow down the absorption rate of sugars and carbohydrates from the intestines into the bloodstream, you don't get blood glucose "spikes." As well as leading to healthier levels of glucose and insulin, whole grains can offer protection for the rest of the body—including prevention of constipation, lowered cholesterol levels, and a reduced chance of dangerous blood clotting.

Nutrition experts now know that we need *both* kinds of fiber—soluble and insoluble. Both are abundantly available in grain foods. Soluble fiber is found primarily in oatmeal, barley, and fruits, while insoluble fiber is common in whole-wheat varieties of breads, cereals, crackers, and many vegetables.

Consumption of whole grains has also been associated with lower rates of several types of cancer, including breast, colon, esophageal, gallbladder, lung, oral, ovarian, prostate, and stomach. It's the entire whole-grain package that con-

(continued . . .)

tributes to the fighting of cancer cells, not the fiber alone. Whole grains possess powerful immune system–boosting antioxidants and many other phytonutrients.

Westerners tend to think of grains as a breakfast food, but if you're smart, you include whole grains throughout the day, in soups, bakery items, and desserts.

Of all the whole grains, oats lead the bunch. Rice is also on the menu every day for more than two billion people on the planet. Whole-grain rice is best. Pasta and couscous are available in whole-grain varieties. Barley is a mild-flavored, kernel-shaped whole grain widely known for its success as a thickening additive in stews and soups.

One of the amazing things about some of the widely touted high-protein diets is the advice to cut out certain good and healthful foods. When you start off on the Atkins Diet, for instance, you're not allowed to eat rice or any grains, absolutely no fruit, no nuts, and no legumes! But you *are* allowed to stuff yourself with protein and lots and lots of animal fat! How crazy is that?

Because rice is readily available, is rich in nutrients, and is a staple of those healthy Okinawans, make it an important part of your meal plans. Whenever possible, substitute brown rice for white rice. Brown rice is less refined and contains more vitamins and more fiber. If you're in a hurry, quick-cooking brown rice will suffice. However, you can cook up a batch of brown rice and store it in a container for a couple of days. Brown rice cooks in water or broth—twice as much liquid as white rice—and it needs to simmer for a full 45 minutes.

The following recipe dresses up plain brown rice with additional ingredients that are good for you:

Brown Rice and Vegetables

Serves 4

    1 cup sliced carrots

    1 tablespoon vegetable oil

    1 cup sliced spring onions

    2 cups cored and chopped apples

    3 cups cooked brown rice

    ½ teaspoon salt

    ½ cup seedless raisins

    1 tablespoon sesame seeds

In a large skillet, over medium heat, sauté the carrots in oil for about five minutes.

Add onions and apples. Cook three to five minutes longer.

Stir in rice, salt, raisins, and sesame seeds. Continue cooking until thoroughly heated.

Other Superfoods from Around the World

As we consider eating habits around the world, the peculiarities of certain regions are noteworthy. For instance, the Mediterranean reliance on monounsaturated fats, such as olive oil, is well documented. There is some protective influence against heart disease and cancer in that diet.

Similarly, the "French paradox" poses a mystery. The French eat quite a lot of fatty food but have a surprisingly low incidence of heart disease. Perhaps it's not a mystery after all—the combination of red wine consumption and lovemaking may do the trick!

Alcohol in moderation can raise your "good" cholesterol level, thereby helping your heart, and that is thanks in part to the chemical resveratrol in red wine. This compound also comes in non-alcoholic foods, including red grapes, purple grapes, and dried raisins that are not sun-dried.

Quercetin, a plant-derived flavonoid, is found in red wine, red and yellow onions, broccoli, and yellow squash.

Japanese green tea is a winner. This tea has antioxidant properties. The Japanese regularly add the jasmine flower to it.

The Eskimos are heavy on the omega-3 oils, which seem to do everything. These oils, as noted earlier, come in cold-water fish. Flaxseeds and flaxseed oil are also rich in omega-3s. They can help thin the blood, lower cholesterol, and reduce inflammation, and they may help reduce arthritic pain and asthmatic reactions. They can possibly reduce the risk of bowel cancer as well.

I know I've missed out on naming lots of miracle foods you've heard about, but this is a good sampling. Notice how none of these super goodies is in meat or cheese, fast foods, or any other Bonus Foods? They seem to hang around in Basic Foods. Funny about that.

||||||||||||||||||||||||||||||||||||||||||||||||||||||||||||||||||||||||||||||||||||||||||||||||||||||||||||||

Chapter 8

Beans

Of all the foods in the world available to humankind, there is none better than beans for good health and an amazing range of tastes.

Bush-type beans are beans, peas are beans, and legumes are beans. On the list of superfoods, beans are right up there at the top. If there's a food that can help you live longer, it's beans.

If you wish to lower your cholesterol, manage (or prevent) diabetes, and boost your vitamin and mineral intake . . . go for beans.

So why don't we eat more of them? Why, in Western societies, don't we eat enough of them to make a difference to our health?

Simple answer: ignorance. We have this peculiar idea that we have to eat lots of red meat to get protein into our bodies. Unless we live in Asia or some Latin American or Mediterranean country, where beans are a staple food, few of us know what kind of beans to buy, nor do we know how to prepare them. Furthermore, we don't know about all the great bean recipes available.

I'm going to help you change that. I'm going to explain why beans are the best food you can eat and what varieties you can buy—or grow—as well as how to prepare and cook them. Recipes love beans, as you'll see from the selection interspersed throughout this chapter.

Are Beans That Good?

Well, beans did rate a mention in the Bible—in the book of Daniel in the Old Testament.

In the sixth century BC—so says the biblical account—a king who had plundered a city in another land captured some of the conquered people and, as an experiment, fed them only vegetables and beans for three years, instead of feeding them meat and wine.

When the prisoners finally stood before the king three years later, he found them 10 times better off than all the magicians and astrologers in his entire realm. The king was Nebuchadnezzar, ruler of Babylon, and the city he besieged and conquered was Jerusalem. Daniel, of course, was the prophet who braved the lion's den and came out unscathed—and he became renowned as the wisest man in the kingdom of Nebuchadnezzar.

Here's another shout-out for beans. In *The Perfumed Garden*, an Arabian fantasy, Sheik Nefzawi gave credit to chickpeas for an incredible display of manliness by Abu el-Heidja, who had apparently made multiple conquests in one frenzied evening of lovemaking "because he surfeited himself with chickpeas . . . and he had drunk camel's milk with honey mixed."

Greek Bean Soup (Fassoulada)

Serves 6–8

>   1 pound dried navy beans, soaked overnight
>
>   1 large onion, peeled and roughly chopped
>
>   3 carrots, sliced
>
>   3 sticks celery, sliced and strings removed
>
>   1 small chili, seeded
>
>   3 large tomatoes, peeled, seeded, and roughly chopped;
>   or 1 can (14.5 ounces) peeled tomatoes, chopped
>
>   2 tablespoons tomato paste
>
>   5 tablespoons olive oil
>
>   Salt and pepper to taste, preferably freshly ground

Drain the soaked beans and place them in a large saucepan.

Cover the beans with cold water and bring it to a boil, skimming off any froth.

Add the onion, carrots, celery, chili, tomatoes, tomato paste, and olive oil and simmer for 1½ hours, or until the beans are tender.

Let cool slightly. Then season with salt and pepper and serve.

Modern Science and Beans

Beans have a powerful history. Here's a modern-day postscript to back up that history.

Under the auspices of the International Union of Nutritional Sciences and the World Health Organization, scientists from Australia, Sweden, Indonesia, and Japan reported in June 2004 on the results of a seven-year study of 785 people age 70 and over from five ethnic groups—Japanese, Swedes, Greeks in Greece,

Greeks in Australia, and Anglo-Celts in Australia. The objective was to identify foods that increased life span.

Legumes (beans and peas) were the only food that crossed cultural differences to increase life span regardless of ethnic background. The scientists at the IUNC and the WHO have concluded: "The study shows that a higher legume intake is the most protective dietary predictor of survival amongst the elderly, regardless of their ethnicity. Legumes have been associated with long-living food cultures such as the Japanese (soy, tofu, natto, miso), the Swedes (brown beans, peas) and the Mediterranean people (lentils, chickpeas, white beans)."

Incidentally, the study also found that higher intakes of mono-unsaturated fats, as reflected in intake of olive oil in Mediterranean cultures, appeared to be protective against premature death, irrespective of one's ethnic background within the Mediterranean region. The takeaway? Use olive oil in your cooking.

Fish was also given a big tick. Fish and shellfish intakes were shown to prolong survival: the study found that this appeared to be related to certain food cultures that have a high intake of fish, such as the Japanese.

Now back to beans. There's also a simple medical reason that beans are good for you—or rather, multiple reasons. Beans are a great source of protein. Beans are high in fiber, which is good for the intestines and for controlling cholesterol. They're also low in calories and fat—and they're good for diabetics because of the balance of complex carbohydrates and proteins. Beans' slowly absorbed carbohydrates provide a steady source of blood glucose and energy. Finally, beans are a great source of B-complex vitamins, iron, potassium, and zinc.

Hearty Lentil Stew

Serves 8

 1 cup dried lentils

 4 cups vegetable stock

 1 pound tomatoes, peeled and diced

 1 large onion, diced

 1 carrot, sliced

 1 large apple, peeled, cored, and diced

 ½ cup frozen peas

 3 cloves garlic, crushed

 1 tablespoon olive oil

 4 tablespoons bottled barbecue sauce

 1 teaspoon paprika

 Salt and pepper to taste

Place the lentils and stock in a large pot.

Bring to a boil; then reduce the heat to low and simmer
 for 20 minutes.

Add the tomatoes, onion, carrot, apple, peas, garlic,
 olive oil, barbecue sauce, and paprika to the pot and
 stir the mixture.

After the soup has simmered for an additional 20 minutes,
 season with salt and pepper and serve.

Full of Beans

Have you ever stopped to think where the saying "He's full of
beans" comes from? What does it mean? It describes a person who
is full of energy. It's no coincidence that the word "bean" is inter-

changeable with "energy" in that saying, because that's exactly what a wide range of beans gives you.

Go to the market—a *real* market—and seek out all the wonderful varieties; then buy some, take them home, cook them, and eat them!

Even a little can of prepared baked beans is a fabulous snack . . . hot or cold, it doesn't matter.

History shows that as nations become wealthier, the intake of red meat increases and the consumption of beans drops alarmingly—to the detriment of our health. A great pity. More vegetable protein and less animal protein is the way to go.

Five-Bean Soup with Ham Hocks

½ cup soybeans

½ cup black beans

½ cup black-eyed peas

½ cup red beans

½ cup white beans

1 pound meaty ham hocks

5 cups water

1 bay leaf

1 cup chicken stock

1 cup diced onion

1 garlic clove, crushed

½ teaspoon thyme

¼ teaspoon pepper

½ teaspoon red pepper flakes

¼ teaspoon Worcestershire sauce

1 can (14.5 ounces) peeled tomatoes, chopped

1 medium carrot, grated

Place beans together in a large saucepan. Cover them with
    2 inches of water and soak them overnight.

Drain water, then add ham hocks, 5 cups water, and the bay leaf.

Simmer, covered, for 1½ hours.

Remove and discard ham hocks, leaving any loose meat.

Add chicken stock, onion, garlic, thyme, pepper, red pepper flakes,
    Worcestershire sauce, tomatoes, and carrot. Cover and simmer
    for 45 minutes.

Add water as needed.

Serve with hot bread.

||||||||||||||||||||||||||||||||||||||||||||||||||||||||||||||||||||||||||||||||||||||||||||||||||||||||||||||||

Chapter 9

Eight Fail-Safe Love, Laugh, and Eat Snacks

I get asked all the time, "Doctor, is there a way to stop being hungry?" My first answer is that when your brain tells you you're hungry, more than half the time you're actually thirsty. So oftentimes a glass of water will do the trick. We often read that we're supposed to drink eight glasses of water a day, though nobody seems to know which authority told us to do that. Asian villagers who live into their 90s don't drink water out of plastic bottles. And they've probably never heard about the eight-glass rule! They get their hydration primarily from Basic Foods.

It's your tongue that causes most of the trouble. Your brain and your stomach will tell you when you're hungry, and they're usually easily satiated—particularly your stomach. It doesn't care what you put into it as long as it's fed three or four times a day. But your taste buds, which are located on the front one-sixth of your tongue, are tiny little tyrants. They're never satisfied. They crave sugar, salt, and fat because you've trained them to crave those things. Because there are no taste buds in your head or in your stomach, you're really feeding only your tongue when you go back for your fourth or fifth piece of chocolate.

‖‖‖

TICKELL TIP

Bad food is packed with fat to make it taste good. But bad food benefits only the tip of your tongue. Good food, on the other hand, benefits the entire body. Once you start eating good food, you'll start to look slimmer, feel better, think more clearly, and attract more people.

‖‖‖

Most so-called diet plans say you don't need snacks as long as you eat heaps of protein with your main meal. I strongly disagree with this approach. There's nothing wrong with snacking. Humans have always eaten whenever they find food.

You shouldn't starve yourself all day, then devour huge, unhealthful meals to satisfy your appetite. The trick is to eat healthful, satisfying, and delicious snacks whenever you're hungry. I've come up with a list of eight Fail-Safe Snacks that are guaranteed to kill your hunger. Try a Fail-Safe Snack whenever you're genuinely hungry—but not just because you're passing the fridge or feeling anxious or sad.

Generally speaking, there are three snack times per day: morning, afternoon, and evening. Again, though: eat a snack only if you're truly hungry between meals. Remember, when it comes to your appetite, snacks always fill the cracks.

1. A spoonful of low-fat yogurt

2. A few sips of a Simple Smoothie (recipe below)

3. A cup of vegetable or minestrone soup

4. A few sardines or half a small can of tuna on a half slice of whole-grain toast

5. Half a banana spread on a half slice of whole-grain toast

6. A few unsalted nuts (almonds, walnuts, soy nuts)

7. A spoonful of hummus on a half slice of whole-grain toast

8. Half a can of baked beans—minus the sauce—on a half slice of whole-grain toast

Simple Smoothie

2 cups soy and/or skim milk

A few spoonfuls of low-fat yogurt

Any fruits: banana, mango, berries, peach, etc.

1 teaspoon honey (optional)

A few drops vanilla extract

Blend and enjoy! Refrigerate any leftover smoothie.

||||||||||||||||||||||||||||||||||||||||||||||||||||||||||||||||||||||||||||||||||||||||||||||||||||||||||||||||||||||||||||||||

Chapter 10

Meal Plans That Work

If you're too busy to spend a lifetime searching out the ultimate diet program, let me offer a few ideas that might help move your meal planning toward the healthier side. Think back on the main food lessons we've covered so far: eating for health means, in a nutshell, favoring Basic Foods over Bonus Foods and avoiding foods that have a high human interference (HI) index.

Fortunately, eating well doesn't mean going hungry. When you eat Basic Foods, you can eat a lot *more* food. That's partly because you're eating a lot fewer calories. A lump of fatty meat contains up to four times the calories of a bunch of vegetables that are roughly the same portion size.

In this chapter I offer three meal plans that introduce you to eating the Love, Laugh, and Eat way. These plans will help you determine what to eat to ensure that you're getting enough calories and nutrients—in short, that you're eating right—without throwing calories away on junk. You can choose whichever plan appeals to you, or work your way through them one by one to get a feel for the Love, Laugh, and Eat program.

Plan 1: Dr. John's Banana Buster Plan

Bananas are an instant-energy, natural food. They're easy to carry, easy to eat; they have lots of fiber, B group vitamins, and potassium. They're good for your intestines and bowel function, and they're already packed and ready to go! They're great for children as well. To get the maximum benefit from this plan, including weight loss, follow these guidelines five to seven days per week for three weeks. If you're already feeling good and just want to maintain your current health and eating habits, follow the guidelines three or four days a week.

Drink two glasses of water before every meal over the course of this plan.

Breakfast

Two pieces of whole-grain toast. No butter, margarine, or salt. Add slices of tomato and pepper to taste.

Or

A small bowl of whole-grain cereal plus fresh fruit and low-fat milk.

No lunch (but remember that between-meal snacks are just fine).

Dinner

Three to four ounces of fish, lean meat, or chicken breast minus the skin. At least three vegetables, preferably dark green (broccoli, spinach, peas), yellow or orange (carrots, pumpkin), and white (potato, cauliflower, cabbage). Make sure, too, that you're getting enough cruciferous vegetables, including cauliflower, cabbage, broccoli, brussels sprouts, and bok choy. Remember that cruciferous vegetables are packed with phytochemicals, some of which are major cancer fighters.

Snacks

Choose from the following snacks between meals—basically any time you're truly hungry.

Half a banana and two glasses of water. A reasonable maximum, over the course of the day, is eight half bananas or four whole bananas. (This *is* the Banana Buster Plan, after all!) Squash or mash the banana on a piece of whole-grain bread if you wish. Just don't use any butter or margarine.

Or

One oat-bran muffin and two glasses of water.

Or

One low-calorie rice cake.

Avoid alcohol on Banana Buster days. Tea and coffee are allowed, but no more than two cups per day (*not* lattes or cappuccinos).

Plan 2: Dr. John's Three-Week VFCF Meal Plan

VFCF stands for vegetables/fruit/chicken/fish. Those foods are your focus over the three weeks of this plan. Rather than laying out each meal, let's look at the basic dos and don'ts of VFCF:

Dos

You may eat *any* fruits, vegetables, and salads, excluding avocado and olives.

Feel free to enjoy either skinless chicken breast or fish, but no more than seven meals per week.

For breakfast, eat some fresh fruit and one or two pieces of whole-grain bread or toast spread with banana, tomato, or cooked asparagus. Skip the margarine, but pepper and a slim scrape of avocado would be okay.

Don'ts

No added salt.

No oils. Try vinegar and/or lemon juice as a dressing.

No cooking in fat. Instead, grill, broil, boil, steam, or microwave. You can also pan-fry in a nonstick pan. A wok is a great alternative.

No red meat.

Apart from skim or low-fat milk, no dairy foods, including butter and margarine, cheese, and eggs.

No cereal. Certain cereals, including muesli, are quite healthful, but they're also high in calories. Many contain dried fruits and coconut, which up the calorie count. During this three-week meal plan, grains are better eaten via a couple pieces of whole-grain toast or bread with some tomato, asparagus, or banana.

No butter or margarine on bread or toast, but a touch of olive oil is fine if you wish.

Fluids

Tap water, soda water, and mineral water. No tonic water.

Two glasses of water before every meal.

Black coffee or green tea. No sugar. Sweeteners such as stevia are okay. A dribble of milk if you must. Green tea is best.

Alcohol, if you wish—preferably wine—but only one day per week, and one or two glasses only.

No fruit juice. Eat the fruit instead.

Vitamins

If this meal plan is a marked departure from your normal eating habits, I suggest taking a multivitamin supplement every day.

Snacks

Have a Fail-Safe Snack (see chapter 9) whenever you're genuinely hungry.

Enjoy fresh fruits or lightly cooked or raw vegetables when mealtime feels too far away.

A great way to snack at the office is to pop some cut-up vegetables into a plastic bag before you leave home. Keep it handy in your office desk drawer. If you get hungry, nibble on veggie chunks and drink some water with ice, topped with a slice or two of lemon.

One Day's Suggested Menu

Two glasses of water before every meal.

Breakfast: Fruit, tea, and toast with tomato and pepper to taste.

Lunch: Salad, or lettuce and tomato sandwich, or salmon sandwich, or tuna fish sandwich, served with tomato and optional cottage cheese.

> *If you eat out for lunch or dinner, order grilled fish with a side of vegetables or a small salad. No sauce or dressing—though if you must, order it on the side.*

Dinner: Lightly cooked vegetables with a portion of fish or chicken breast.

Dessert: Fruit with perhaps a touch of low-fat yogurt.

Plan 3: Dr. John's In the Soup Plan

This is the best plan to use if you're trying to break through a weight-loss plateau or halt a rise in weight.

Follow this plan for three weeks, or for however long you want to continue.

Be sure to drink two glasses of water before every meal with this plan.

Breakfast

Tea and two pieces of whole-grain toast with banana or sliced tomato. No butter or margarine or salt.

> *Or*

A small bowl of whole-grain cereal with some fresh fruit and low-fat milk.

Lunch

Green salad topped with salmon or tuna fish.

   Or

A three-ounce portion of fish or lean meat or skinless chicken breast plus vegetables or salad with lemon and vinegar.

   Or

Pasta dish with a tomato-based sauce.

Dinner

After 2:00 P.M., nothing but vegetable soup. You can try other soups every now and again, but vegetable soup works best and is the best for you. If you wish, make a minestrone soup with as many different vegetables as you can find, adding just a touch of pasta or rice.

Snacks

More soup. Yup—soup for snack! Don't forget to take some homemade vegetable soup to the office with you.

Once a week reward yourself with a glass or two of wine. But no beer. Three things about beer: (1) a glass of beer contains more fluid than a glass of wine; (2) folks usually can't stop after a single glass of beer; and while wine—red wine, in particular—contains antioxidants, beer contains hardly any.

Chapter 11

IIIIIIIIIIIIIIIIIIIIIIIIIIIIIIIIIIIIIIIIIIIIIIIIIIIIIIIIIIIIIIIIIIIIIIIIIIIIIIIIIIIII

The Seven-Day Love, Laugh, and Eat Cleanse

*G*iven how polluted our air, water, and soil are, and how much fast food most Americans consume, it's not surprising that we end up full of toxins and poisons. A periodic cleanse is a good way to get rid of some of those toxins. I recommend a seven-day cleanse before you begin any of the meal plans in the previous chapter, and perhaps twice a year thereafter.

There are two ways to cleanse your body. One is a virtual starvation, which entails consuming only some herbal teas and pure juices. I'm against this approach. I believe that the best way to restart your body is to go right back to the basics by taking in only simple fruits and vegetables for three days. Then, after the initial cleanse, reintroduce into your diet simple and wholesome foods, as shown below.

[Day 1]

Breakfast

Glass of water with lemon slice

A variety of slices of fruit (equivalent to one piece of fruit)

Grilled tomatoes and bok choy; no salt, but pepper okay

Cup of green or jasmine tea

Snacks

Glass of water with lemon slice

One Fail-Safe Snack (page 159)

Lunch

Glass of water with lemon slice

Vegetarian Miso Soup

Vegetarian Miso Soup

Serves 3

    1½ tablespoons miso paste
    2½ cups vegetable stock
    8 fresh shiitake mushrooms
    2 ounces firm tofu, cut into half-inch cubes
    1 small carrot, finely shredded
    1 small white radish, finely shredded
    2 spring onions (using both green portion and white),
        finely chopped

Combine the miso paste with the vegetable stock
    and heat through.

Add the whole shiitake mushrooms and simmer the mixture as you cut up the remaining ingredients.

Add the tofu, carrot, and radish to the simmering soup base and cook for one to two minutes more.

Sprinkle spring onions in bowls. Pour the soup over the onions and serve.

Dinner

Glass of water with lemon slice

Vegetarian Miso Soup (page 170)

Evening Snack

Two spoonfuls of low-fat yogurt or a sip of Simple Smoothie (page 159) or a small cup of vegetable soup

[Day 2]

Breakfast

Glass of water with lemon slice

A variety of slices of fruit (equivalent to one piece of fruit)

Grilled tomatoes and bok choy; no salt, but pepper okay

Cup of green or jasmine tea

[Breakfast: Break the Fast]

Breakfast used to be two separate words: "break" and "fast." Those two words still function in "breakfast," which *breaks* the roughly 17-hour *fast* between dinner last night and lunch today.

Breakfast is particularly important for those of us who are rolling along into that Dangerous Decade—the decade from 44 to 54—when responsible people under tremendous pressure start to fall to bits. Things fall out, things fall off, things go into spasm.

Most of us eat all our food between the hours of 1:00 and 8:00 P.M., stuffing our faces during those hours, then abstaining for the next 17, save for the occasional coffee or cigarette to kick-start the motor.

Which is why breakfast isn't just breakfast; it's a *break* to this *fast*.

If you *don't* break the 17-hour fast, you're playing a risky game. The risks include lower energy to start the day. Unclear thinking. An insatiable craving for sugary, fatty pick-me-up foods. A higher risk of diabetes and of bowel cancer, to name just a few.

Preparing and eating breakfast takes about four minutes every morning. Those four minutes are, arguably, the most important four minutes of your day. Breakfast gets everything moving and sets you up for a good beginning. Four minutes, that's it. "Can't afford four minutes, Doctor. I don't have the time. Besides, I don't feel hungry." Rubbish. Go to bed four minutes earlier the night before.

Now, what's best for breakfast? Variety is good, especially when you're choosing among fruits, *whole* grains, and fiber.

And we can learn from our Asian friends, who usually add small amounts of fish, beans, and rice.

Remember that we're shooting for the Rule of 15. Breakfast is a great opportunity to put at least half a dozen different plant foods—those Basic Foods—on your scoreboard.

If you're going to eat packaged cereals, be careful. The food labeling laws in the United States are pretty good, but those in most other Western countries aren't so good. Be wary of excess sugars, refined products, and trans fats (which I warned about in chapter 3).

Muesli—either store-bought or homemade—is a wonderful alternative to cereal. Add some low-fat yogurt, skim milk, or soy milk. It tastes great and it's great for you.

It takes only four minutes a day to reduce your risk of developing colon cancer. You get your intestines moving with fiber after they've been asleep! Science is telling us that, so why wouldn't you do it?

TICKELL TIP

You *must* have fiber at breakfast time. Fiber is the roughage that fills you up and helps to sweep the nasty toxins and poisons through your intestines and *out the back door!* Fiber is found only in Basic Foods (vegetables, fruits, grains, nuts, and seeds)—natural foods that haven't been interfered with by human beings. There is no fiber in sausages, bacon, and eggs!

Snacks

Glass of water with lemon slice

One Fail-Safe Snack (page 159)

Lunch

Glass of water with lemon slice

Vegetarian Miso Soup (page 170)

Dinner

Glass of water with lemon slice

Vegetarian Miso Soup (page 170)

Evening Snack

Two spoonfuls of low-fat yogurt or a sip of Simple Smoothie (page 159) or a small cup of vegetable soup

[Day 3]

Breakfast

Glass of water with lemon slice

A variety of slices of fruit (equivalent to one piece of fruit)

Grilled tomatoes and bok choy; no salt, but pepper okay

Cup of green or jasmine tea

Lunch

Glass of water with lemon slice

Vegetarian Miso Soup (page 170)

Snacks

Fail-Safe Snacks (but only if required; page 159), midmorning, midafternoon, and evening

Dinner

Glass of water with lemon slice

Spicy Steamed Sea Bass and Broccoli

Spicy Steamed Sea Bass and Broccoli

Serves 2

- ⅔ pound sea bass fillets
- Black pepper
- 3 spring onions, sliced
- 2 red chilies, seeded and chopped; additional for garnish if you wish
- 1 clove garlic, chopped
- ½-inch piece fresh ginger root, grated
- 4 tablespoons light soy sauce
- 4 tablespoons Chinese white wine (optional)
- 2 tablespoons chopped cilantro
- 1 head broccoli, cut into bite-size pieces and steamed separately

Carefully remove bones from the sea bass. Season the fillets with pepper and let them sit for two to three minutes as you prepare the vegetables.

Mix the onions, chilies, garlic, and ginger with the soy sauce and wine.

Spoon that mixture over the fish and place in a
   steamer over heat; continue steaming until the
   fish is cooked through.

Remove from the steamer and place on a serving
   plate. Sprinkle with cilantro (and extra chilies, if
   desired).

Serve with steamed broccoli.

[Day 4]

Breakfast

Glass of water with lemon slice

A variety of slices of fruit (equivalent to one piece of fruit)

Egg-White Frittata

Egg-White Frittata

Serves 6

   ½ onion, chopped
   ½ cup green pepper, chopped
   ½ cup red pepper, chopped
   ½ cup spinach, chopped
   15 medium mushrooms, sliced
   5 medium tomatoes, chopped
   2 spring onions, chopped
   ½ bunch fresh basil
   Black pepper
   16 eggs, separated; use whites only

In a nonstick pan, sauté the onion, green pepper,
   and red pepper with a little water until softened.

Add the spinach, mushrooms, and tomatoes and cook briefly.

Add the spring onions and fresh basil and season to taste with the black pepper. Allow the mixture to cool completely.

Lightly beat the egg whites, then mix with the vegetable medley.

Heat a small nonstick skillet and pour in the mix, as if making a pancake. Cook over medium heat until the mixture is set. Then, with extreme care, flip the frittata to cook the other side. Alternatively, place the pan under the broiler to cook the top of the frittata.

Lunch

Glass of water with lemon slice

Vegetarian Miso Soup (page 170)

Dinner

Chinese-Style Stir-Fried Veal

Chinese-Style Stir-Fried Veal

Serves 4

1 pound veal loin
3 spring onions, sliced
½ medium onion, chopped
2 cloves garlic, minced
1-inch piece fresh ginger root, peeled and grated
2 ounces dried shiitake mushrooms, soaked and sliced
1 small red chili, seeded (unless you want extra zip) and finely chopped

2 tablespoons white wine
1½ tablespoons soy sauce
1 tablespoon cornstarch
¾ cup vegetable stock
2 cups steamed brown rice

Trim and slice the veal into thin slices, then put back into the refrigerator.

Because this meal goes together quickly, arrange in separate small bowls the prepared spring onions, medium onion, garlic, ginger, shiitake mushrooms, and chili.

In another bowl, whisk together the wine, soy sauce, and cornstarch.

Heat a wok or large skillet over medium-high heat until hot. Add the onions (both types), garlic, and ginger and toss them. Add about 2 tablespoons of the vegetable stock and stir in. Continue to stir and add, in the following order, shiitake mushrooms, veal, remaining vegetable stock, and chili.

Once the stock starts to evaporate a little and the color begins to brown, gradually add the cornstarch mix, stirring the contents of the wok to avoid lumps. This should thicken the liquid so that it coats the back of a spoon.

Remove into a serving dish and serve with the steamed brown rice.

Snacks

Morning, afternoon, and evening as required

[Day 5]

Breakfast

Glass of water with lemon slice

A variety of slices of fruit (equivalent to one piece of fruit)

Grilled tomatoes and bok choy; no salt, but pepper okay

Cup of green or jasmine tea

Lunch

Stir-Fried Thai Rice Noodles

Stir-Fried Thai Rice Noodles

Serves 6

- 1 cup snow peas
- 1 large carrot, cut into thin strips
- 1 cup baby corn, cut in half lengthwise
- 1 cup kale, roughly chopped
- ½ cup vegetable stock (or as required)
- ½ medium onion, finely chopped
- 6 cloves garlic, crushed
- 6 large fresh chilies (or to taste), seeded and finely chopped
- 1 pound rice noodles, cooked
- 4 teaspoons soy sauce
- 1 cup Thai basil leaves

Blanch the snow peas, carrot, corn, and kale in boiling water.

Plunge them into cold water to chill; drain well and set aside.

In a wok or large nonstick frying pan, pour a little of the vegetable stock and add the onion and garlic. Cook until the onion is transparent and almost dry, adding a little extra stock if the mix becomes too dry.

Carefully pull the rice noodles apart and add to the wok or pan.

Toss well, adding a little extra vegetable stock as necessary.

Add the cooked vegetables and chilies to taste.

Toss well to heat through.

Season with soy sauce and add the basil leaves. Mix well and serve.

Dinner

Tuna Steak with Tomato and Salad

Tuna Steak with Tomato and Salad

Serves 4

   4 3½-ounce tuna steaks
   Salt substitute
   4 tomatoes
   4 spring onions, finely chopped
   3⅓ tablespoons apple cider vinegar
   2 tablespoons apple juice concentrate
   3 shallots, finely chopped
   1 tablespoon soy sauce
   1 to 2 tablespoons vegetable stock (optional)
   4 cups lettuce leaves, ripped into bite-size pieces
   ½ cup chopped cilantro

Season tuna steaks heavily with salt substitute on both sides.

Cut the tomatoes in half and discard the seeds. Dice the flesh.

In a small bowl, combine the tomatoes, spring onions, vinegar, apple concentrate, shallots, and soy sauce. Set aside.

In a very hot nonstick pan, sear the tuna steaks, adding a little vegetable stock if the tuna looks too dry.

Arrange the lettuce on a serving plate, top with the seared tuna, and spoon the sauce over both the fish and lettuce.

Decorate liberally with the cilantro and serve.

[Day 6]

Breakfast

Glass of water with lemon slice

A variety of slices of fruit (equivalent to one piece of fruit)

Egg-White Frittata (see recipe, page 176: adapt by including 1 egg yolk for every 4 egg whites if you wish)

Lunch

Seafood Miso Soup

Seafood Miso Soup

Serves 4

1½ tablespoons miso paste
2½ cups vegetable stock

4 fresh shiitake mushrooms
2 ounces firm tofu, cut into ½-inch cubes
1 small carrot, finely shredded
1 small daikon white radish, finely shredded
¼ pound prawns, peeled
¼ pound snapper fillet, cut into chunks
2 spring onions, chopped

Prepare as for Vegetarian Miso Soup, but add the
    prawns and snapper when you add the tofu
    and vegetables to the simmering soup base
    and cook for two to three minutes.

Serve over spring onions as for the Vegetarian
    Miso Soup.

_____

Dinner

Chicken with Nori and Herbs

_____

Chicken with Nori and Herbs

Serves 4

4 skinless chicken breasts (about 1 pound total)
2 sheets nori seaweed
1 tablespoon soy sauce
1 ice cube
1 tablespoon salt substitute
1 large carrot, cut into chunks
8 pieces baby corn, cut into chunks
2 zucchini, cut into chunks
Scant ¼ pound snow peas, halved
½ cup vegetable stock
2 tablespoons chopped parsley

Place 1 chicken breast in a food processor with the
    nori, the soy sauce, and the ice cube. Pulse-blend
    until almost smooth.

Cut a pocket into each of the remaining chicken breasts and fill with the nori mix. Sprinkle with salt substitute and refrigerate until needed.

Cook the prepared carrot, corn, zucchini, and snow peas in a steamer.

Heat a heavy-based pan and add a little of the vegetable stock. When hot, add the chicken breasts. Continue to cook on medium heat for five to eight minutes, adding a little extra vegetable stock if the pan becomes too dry. Do not overcook the chicken.

To serve, arrange the vegetables and chicken on a serving plate, spoon over a few drops of cooking juice from the pan, and sprinkle with chopped parsley.

[**Day 7**]

Breakfast

Glass of water with lemon slice

A variety of slices of fruit (equivalent to one piece of fruit)

Grilled tomatoes and bok choy; no salt, but pepper okay

Cup of green or jasmine tea

Lunch

Tempeh Salad (page 184)

Tempeh Salad

Serves 4

- ⅓ pound tempeh, thinly sliced
- 2 large carrots, grated
- 2 turnips, grated
- 2 beets, grated and cooked
- 2 teaspoons sesame seeds
- 3 tablespoons apple cider vinegar
- 1 sheet nori seaweed, sliced into fine strips

Place the tempeh slices in a heated nonstick pan. Fry on both sides without any oil; then remove from pan.

Arrange a row of each of the grated vegetables—carrots, turnips, beets—on a serving plate.

Arrange the warm tempeh on top and sprinkle with sesame seeds and apple cider vinegar. Garnish with strips of nori.

Tip: If the tempeh sticks to the pan when you fry it, the pan is not hot enough.

Dinner

Pink Salmon and Vegetables

Now that you have some Asian influence ideas, prepare to your liking 3 to 4 ounces of salmon for each person, plus 5 or 6 vegetables of your choice.

Dessert

Banana "Ice Cream" with Berries

Banana "Ice Cream" with Berries

Serves 6

> 6 bananas
> 1 pint blueberries
> 1 pint strawberries, trimmed and halved
> Shaved dark chocolate (optional)

Peel the bananas and place in a plastic bag, then freeze.

About two hours before serving, place the frozen bananas in a food processor and puree.

Transfer the puree to a metal container and return it to the freezer for about two hours, or until firm.

Remove the banana "ice cream" from the freezer 10 to 15 minutes before serving. Spoon about half into chilled glass dishes and top with a layer of blueberries, then strawberries, then blueberries, then strawberries, then blueberries again; top with remaining banana "ice cream."

Sprinkle with the shaved chocolate (if using) and serve immediately.

Chapter 12

||||||||||||||||||||||||||||||||||||||||||||||||||||||||||||||||||||||||||||||||||||||||||||||||||||||

Love, Laugh, and Eat
for Dummies

A s you learn how to Love, Laugh, and Eat, I want to set you up with a few handy tips and guidelines, which will go a long way toward helping you enjoy life as never before. Think of this chapter as the official Love, Laugh, and Eat cheat sheet, your very own Eating for Dummies, the Moderates edition. This really is the pathway to success.

Accountability counts. Remember, you're looking after *you*, the greatest machine on earth. Keeping track of your behavior (and your progress) will keep you on that success pathway and encourage further progress.

Each week, tally your Living*life* points in the Success Chart on page 188. During your Switch On weeks, aim for around 72 of these points. Aim for a minimum of 60 Living*life* points during Hold weeks.

Success Chart

ACE	Week								Living*life* Points		
		M	W	T	F	S	S		My Total	Goal	Max
A1	Did I do my walk today? 2 points per day—goal is 14 points per week *If you walk a minimum of 5 days per week, score 4 bonus points.*								___	14	14
A2	Did I do my strength work today? 1 point per day—goal is 4 or 5 points per week								___	5	7
A3	Did I do my OUMs today? 1 point per day—goal is 4 or 5 points per week								___	5	7
	ACTIVITY TOTALS								___	**24**	**28**
		M	W	T	F	S	S				
C1	Did I laugh and give someone a hug today? 1 point per day—goal is 6 points per week								___	6	7
C2	Did I do some deep breathing and another relaxation thing today? 1 point per day—goal is 6 points per week								___	6	7
C3	Did I sleep well last night? 1 point per day—goal is 6 points per week								___	6	7
C4	Did I do something good for or be nice to someone else today? 1 point per day—goal is 6 points per week								___	6	7
	COPING TOTALS								___	**24**	**28**
		M	W	T	F	S	S				
E1	Did I eat/nibble my 15 plant foods today? 2 points per day—goal is 12 points per week								___	12	14
E2	Did I do the two-thirds/one-third routine today? 1 point per day—goal is 6 points per week								___	6	7
E3	Did I eat breakfast today? 1 point per day—goal is 6 points per week								___	6	7
	EATING TOTALS								___	**24**	**28**
	WEEKLY GRAND TOTAL								___	**72**	**84**

Switch On weeks: Aim for 72 LLPs.
Hold weeks: Why not aim for the same number of LLPs?

Keep track, too, of your activity sessions. Make appointments with yourself, because you are the best personal trainer in the world. Keep up the BAT exercises and the OUMs. Remember that the goal is to keep active for 1 percent of your week, which is 100 minutes every seven days, or four 25-minutes sessions.

||||||||||||||||||||||||||||||||||||||||||||||||||||||||||||||||||||||||||||||||||

TICKELL TIP

Improve your flexibility. Total body flexibility is really important, especially if you tend to get back and/or neck pain. A couple of minutes of stretching and flexibility work can give you a huge payback. Do some stretches before or after your walk and include some back and neck movements regularly, especially if you have an office job or drive a car for long periods of time.

||||||||||||||||||||||||||||||||||||||||||||||||||||||||||||||||||||||||||||||||||

For each activity and meal, give yourself:

- 2 points *each* for walking and for following the Rule of 15
- 1 point *each* for BAT and OUM exercises, for following the Two-Thirds, One-Third Rule at a meal, for eating breakfast, and for each "thing" you do from the Relaxation List

It's really easy and *it works*.

Really Good Ideas

When it comes to dieting, there's no shortage of Really Good Ideas. The problem is figuring out which ones to follow. Here are some of my favorites:

Skip the Supermarket

Instead of heading for the supermarket, go to an *actual* market, a farmers' market. That's where the *really* fresh produce—newly harvested vegetables and fruit—is located, and many such markets also have meat and fish vendors. These markets carry foods that humans haven't had the chance to mess around with. These are the foods that are low in so-called human interference. It's real food; it's good food. It's not plastic or processed food-like stuff. And there are very few labels to confuse you. At an old-fashioned market, there's also no extravaganza of refined junk or cold tantalizing cans of liquid sugar to tempt you on your way to the checkout counter.

A Little Goes a Long Way

Another Really Good Idea is to avoid huge meals. You just don't need them. A great way to fill yourself up before your main meal is to have a small bowl of vegetable soup or miso soup. And remember to drink two glasses of water before every meal. A slice of lemon, combined with that water, will help curb your appetite. Then you'll only have to eat for *two* instead of *three:* while your head and stomach are fed, your tongue can sit this one out.

Snack More with Less

While we're on the subject of the tongue, the best snacks are the ones that satisfy your tongue *and* your stomach but contain very few calories. It's a Really Good Idea to eat these. If your diet book says you don't need snacks, it's probably also telling you to eat lots and lots of meat-based protein meals. Beware! Psychologically, you *do* need snacks.

Some of my favorites include a few sips of skim milk or soy milk or soy smoothie, and/or a couple spoonfuls of low-fat yogurt. I'm not a calorie counter, but I can tell you that what I've just mentioned adds 10 or 20 calories, while just one bite of a chocolate or snack bar can run up to 100 or 200 calories. An entire chocolate bar can run as high as 1,000 calories! And while a small packet of chips is around 500 calories, the big packs contain about 2,500 calories. Wow! That's enough calories for a whole day! It's a Really Good Idea and a Really Simple Idea to skip snacks that are high in calories. When in doubt, try my Fail-Safe Snacks (page 159).

‖‖

TICKELL TIP

One in three Americans will get cancer. Either you or your partner or a good friend or acquaintance will get cancer. Don't want it? Then build your immune system with your ACE skills.

‖‖

Fifteen and Counting

Remember to follow the Rule of 15. This is another Really Good Idea that works astoundingly well, largely because it helps you vary your meals—and, as we all know, variety is the name of the game. Varying your dietary intake gives you more interest, more energy, more brainpower. Don't forget that glucose feeds the brain. And of course if you follow the Rule of 15, you bump up your immune system and decrease your risk of cancer.

Take the Stairs

If you see a bunch of stairs, walk up them—feel your quads and your butt muscles contracting, tightening. Your thighs actually talk to each other and chat about what they've done each day. Give them something good to talk about!

Leave It on the Plate

I hate when people start sentences with "In the old days," but here goes . . .

In the old days, we had nice little cupcakes and muffins. Today, we have gigantic muffins packed with chocolate chips or blueberries—sometimes both—and a million calories. So leave half your muffin on the plate.

Enjoy the occasional treat, but don't feel like you have to eat it *all*. I'm one of the very few people in the world who can go to the minibar in a hotel room, grab a packet of potato chips, eat four chips, and throw the rest in the trash.

"But you've just wasted four dollars," you protest.

No, I've probably just saved my life.

Monitor Portion Size

Do you weigh your food, as advised by some diet plans? Do you have a scale in your kitchen that you use night after night after night when you're preparing your (and your family's) meals? Give it up. There's a better, more interesting way to monitor how much food you eat. It's portion size, not weight.

Take the size of your dinner plate, for instance. What if you ate off smaller plates? If you had a plate that was two-thirds the size of your normal plate, you couldn't pile on as much food. If you ate off smaller plates for three months, you'd lose a lot of pounds of fat.

And what about the size of your palm? A serving of meat should be no bigger than the palm of your hand. It certainly shouldn't be the size of half a cow! By eating portions of meat smaller than (or the same size as) the palm of your hand—3 to 3½ ounces of meat per serving—you will dramatically reduce your risk of developing colon cancer, according to the World Cancer Research Fund.

If you want to risk getting colon cancer in the next 10 years, go ahead and eat half a cow every meal. If you don't want colon cancer, reduce the portion of meat to the size of your palm.

Remember the Two-Thirds, One-Third Rule. A steak isn't supposed to cover the WHOLE plate, just one-third of the plate. Two-thirds of each meal needs to come from Basic Foods—vegetables, grains, salads, etc. A steak should NOT be half a cow!

Finally, what about the size of your fork and knife? In Okinawa, they don't have forks. They have chopsticks. It's very difficult to eat fast with chopsticks, because you can't just shovel food into your mouth. Chopsticks force you to eat slowly, which lets you recognize when your stomach and head are fully satisfied.

Weighing doesn't work, but portion size does.

Do you need the largest coffee? Do you need the coffee *and* the muffin? No, you don't.

Basic Guidelines

In addition to the Really Good Ideas above, I want you to follow a few simple Basic Guidelines as you Love, Laugh, and Eat.

Scales

Get off your bathroom scale. Do you weigh yourself every day? If you do, don't. Once a week is fine. The scale doesn't tell you everything. How do you feel today? Instead of stepping on the scale, slip on your favorite suit or dress every three weeks or so. Does it fit more comfortably? I bet it does. Keep it on and go out with your partner, significant other, or spouse. If you're a male, is it one more notch on your belt—or maybe one less?

Barbecues

Any good? Not too often. Once in a while is fine. Don't burn the meat, though. When you burn and blacken flesh, you produce chemical compounds that can increase the risk of cancer.

Alcohol

For people who enjoy alcohol, there are three levels of alcohol intake, corresponding to their level of desperation. Think about where you might fit on the spectrum:

- *Not desperate.* You don't drink any alcohol during the week, or maybe only a glass of wine during the weekend.

- *Moderately desperate.* You drink one glass of wine with the evening meal four or five times a week.

- *Definitely desperate.* You drink one or two glasses of wine every night of the week, and more on weekends.

||||||||||||||||||||||||||||||||||||||||||||||||||||||||||||||||||||||||||||||||

TICKELL TIP

Almost all businesspeople who routinely drink
alcohol at lunchtime are fat. That's a fact. Stick to soda
water at lunch and limit your alcohol intake to after
the sun goes down. Even then—ask yourself,
Should I have an AFD today?

||||||||||||||||||||||||||||||||||||||||||||||||||||||||||||||||||||||||||||||||

[AFDs]

A little more than a decade ago, I invented AFDs to help people cope with stress and maximize health. An AFD is an alcohol-free day. This is another Really Good Idea.

Many people drink every day of their lives, using alcohol as a crutch. Naturally, their tolerance for alcohol increases. As a result, as time goes by they need more and more and more drinks to achieve the same effect.

If you're prepared to throw in an AFD two or three times a week, you'll learn to keep your alcohol intake at a moderate level. An AFD is a great discipline.

People say they don't want discipline in their lives, but that's not true. We all actually, secretly, love discipline. Discipline rewards us. When business gets a little tough, people need to get tough right back—sharpen their pencils, make hard decisions, tough decisions. This is how people succeed in business. And yet a simple thing like self-management eludes most folks. People in business, effective managers in the workplace, are usually awful at managing *themselves* until they're faced with a crisis or a life-threatening event. Then they suddenly figure out how to do it.

An AFD is a great discipline for everyday drinkers. Your body will love you for it. Put two AFDs together and you can almost hear your liver applaud—sensational. "Thank you very much," your body says. In addition to the sudden accolades, you'll start to sleep better.

Two AFDs a week will significantly cut down on the number of drinks you imbibe every seven days, which will have an immediate and long-term benefit for your body. No hangovers,

(continued . . .)

for one thing—and your body will start to feel younger, healthier, and more vibrant. Dean Martin used to say he felt sorry for nondrinkers because when they wake up in the morning, that's the best they'll feel all day. But we know now that that's not a good thing. Too much alcohol can kill your liver, your brain, and *you*!

Here's a good party trick. If you're in a social situation and the host is constantly trying to fill your glass, don't let him or her. Instead, wait until your glass is completely empty; *then* refill it. This way you stay in control.

At the end of each week—say, every Sunday morning—count up how many drinks you had in the past week. Trust me, this isn't an easy thing to do. It frightens some people. Sometimes people don't even realize that they've consumed 35 or more drinks in seven days until they start doing the math. "Yeah, but that was a bad week," they usually tell me. But then they remember that they drank 40 or 50 drinks the week before.

Not only is it scary, it's also a hell of a lot of calories.

Alcohol kills brain cells and liver cells. That's definitely scary. But a seven-ounce glass of beer, a four-ounce glass of wine, and a one-ounce glass of spirits such as gin or whiskey all contain 70 to 100 calories. So two drinks a night equals 14 drinks a week, which is 1,400 calories. Every three weeks you put on an extra pound. In a year, that's 16 pounds that you have to burn off to stay level. It takes an hour walking to burn up the calories from three drinks—that's five hours walking every week to stay at the same weight. Scary stuff, indeed.

Alcohol is not such a bad drug in moderation, but when taken in excess it can wreck your health and your personal life. Use AFDs to keep it under control.

Fruit Juice

Fresh fruit juice can often be nutritious, but it contains lots of calories. How many oranges do you need to squeeze to end up with a glass of orange juice? Four? Six? During your Switch On periods, skip the juice. Eat the fruit instead.

Soft Drinks, Soda Pop

Soda pop is a huge source of calories in this country, and the diet drinks, while low-cal, are full of chemicals, natural and unnatural. Pop is also highly addictive. We can't get enough of it. The average person today consumes up to 10 times what we used to. This level of exposure messes with your metabolism and screws up your appetite. Once the sugar high ends, you crash and reach out for another soda, constantly craving more pop.

What's wrong with water or a nice cup of tea? Or how about some homemade lemonade? Squeeze half a lemon into a glass of water and add a pinch of unrefined sea salt and a few shavings of ginger root for a healthy and refreshing alternative to sugary soft drinks. If you want the fizz of soda without the calories or the sugar high (and low), a tablespoon of raw apple-cider vinegar, a good probiotic, in a glass of sparkling mineral water should do the trick.

Cereals

In the Switch On weeks, stay clear of cereals in packets, packages, boxes, cartons—everything but the absolute basics, such as whole grains or oats. If you wish to reintroduce small helpings of whole-grain cereals later on, that's okay with me. A homemade muesli mix can be a good idea, but go easy on the serving size; there are lots of calories in dried fruits.

Starch

Bread, potatoes, and pasta are often referred to as "starches." Starch is a no-no according to many diet books. Starch is glucose, which is a pure form of energy, and it burns clean. My belief is that any problem with starch has to do with the level of refinement—that is, the HI index—and the quantity consumed. Whole-grain breads, small potatoes, and a little pasta now and then are all part of the game of life as played by many normal-weighted, long-living people. Quantity is the problem, and the preparation too—deep-frying, say, or the addition of sauces.

Crackers, Cookies

Cheap, low-grade fats are extremely unhealthful in large quantities. Trans fats and partially hydrogenated fats are the worst. These fats are in many baked items, crackers, cookies, and margarine spreads—making this a group of foods you should rarely eat, if ever! They're also often packed with sugar. More calories, more diabetes, less wellness!

Healthy fats are usually found in natural plant-based foods, including avocados, chia seeds, flaxseeds, and nuts, and in wild fish such as salmon and trout.

Instead of cookies and cake, look around for foods that have not, or have hardly, been interfered with by human beings—foods low on the HI index.

Olive Oil

A teaspoon or two of the Mediterranean Magic doesn't go amiss. A teaspoon contains not many calories at all, and it can make a major taste difference to quite a few foods. Olive oil is a healthful and stable monounsaturated fat, which means it helps the body absorb nutrients.

[Pasta]

The good news about pasta is that it's an excellent "opportunity food." By that I mean you can use it to boost the healthful content of what you eat, and you can use it to introduce a wide variety of taste delights as well.

One belief about pasta is that it's a fattening food, too high in sugars and too prone to toppings that are loaded with fats and dietary "baddies." That's true only if you choose the wrong pasta, cook it the wrong way, load too much on the plate, and pour creamy, fat-laden sauce all over everything.

But it's not true if you choose the right pasta and have the right ingredients in the accompanying sauce or salad.

Good pasta—the kind of pasta I will recommend here—is full of the beneficial carbohydrates that are a necessary part of your healthy life. When you eat the kind of pasta I'm about to introduce, the release of complex carbohydrates provides slow, constant energy; the stomach feels full longer, and the body doesn't experience the highs and lows of wildly swinging blood sugar.

Avoid pasta made from white flour and go for whole-grain pasta. It's not hard to find. Look in your local deli, in your health food shop, in your organic food shop, or on the natural food shelves of your supermarket.

Do I hear you say, "But whole-grain pasta doesn't taste as good?"

Think again. Actually, it's the refined white-flour products that lack flavor and texture, because they're made from flour that has had most of the flavor and texture-contributing parts of the grain removed. White-flour products are often jazzed

(continued . . .)

up with lots of additives (mostly sugar, salt, and fat) to give taste. It's definitely not the white flour that's giving the taste.

White flour is what's left after stripping virtually all the nutrients and fiber out of a whole grain of wheat. What you're left with is a lifeless powder that's a perfect binding agent to hold together sugar, sodium, artificial colors, flavors, preservatives, additives, and other chemicals.

In an attempt to replace some of the destroyed nutrients, food manufacturers restore tiny amounts of synthetic nutrients to "fortify" or "enrich" their products. You may read on the label of a spaghetti product that it's an excellent source of, say, eight essential nutrients, seven of which have been added through fortification! This spaghetti lacks any real nutritional value on its own.

Consuming white-flour products can cause blood sugar levels to rise quickly, which triggers the pancreas to release greater amounts of insulin. This, in turn, *lowers* blood sugar levels just as quickly, which activates the hunger response.

Whole-grain flours come with much more flavor, texture, and naturally occurring fats (not to mention greater and more balanced nutrition), so there's much less need for added flavorings.

Advertising has created a perception that white-flour products are "healthy" because they're low in fat, cholesterol, and calories. People who eat heavily processed pasta, bread, rolls, and pretzels in the belief that they're "eating healthy" because these foods are fat-free are on the wrong train. What food manufacturers fail to mention about white-flour products is that they have close to zero nutritional value and can lead to poor health. White-flour products can lead to the very same problems caused by eating too much refined sugar in foods such as crackers, sweets, cakes, carbonated soft drinks, ice cream, and syrups.

Whole-grain pastas can be combined with dairy foods, legumes, meats, fish, and other protein sources to provide all the amino acids needed for a well-balanced meal plan.

To sum up, whole-grain pasta is an excellent source of B-group vitamins, is low in fat, is cholesterol free, and has little or no sodium.

And here's a useful food fact about whole-grain pasta. Beginning a meal with a small-plate food such as whole-grain pasta, and eating it slowly, will lessen your craving for fats during the rest of the meal. You'll start to feel full and won't want as much of the higher-fat foods—or in fact *any* foods. So use a little pasta (with low-fat sauce) to curb overeating. Do what the healthy Mediterraneans do—a *little* pasta is part of a meal, not the whole meal!

Fast Food

Why do you need fast food? You don't. I eat that stuff maybe three or four times a year—when I can't find anything else, like in an American airport. And I usually take only a couple of bites, then throw the rest in the trash.

Don't forget the HI index, which skyrockets in fast food. Ask yourself—is this natural food, or has someone messed it up in the name of "convenience." Less fast food, more slow food.

Dressings

When you're served food in Bonus land, the servers ask, "What kind of dressing do you want with that? Thousand Island, Blue Cheese, Ranch?" If I say, "I don't want dressing, thank you," they look at me with an inquisitive stare, like I'm from Mars. So I say, "I'll have it on the side, thanks"—which puts *me* in control. You need only about one-eighth of the usual dollop of dressing for the same taste sensation. And when you opt for that smaller serving, you're saving another million calories and a 10-mile walk.

Sauces

If a meal comes with a sauce, especially a cream-based sauce or one I've never heard of, I'll say it again—"on the side, please." Remember, you need only a touch of sauce or gravy to satisfy your taste buds.

Water

"Drink 8 or 10 glasses of water a day," they say. "You can't drink too much water," they say. Well, who are "they"? Whoever dreamed up this one was obviously on the crazy high-protein or high-fat bandwagon, because when you're eating mainly plant foods, you're taking in lots of water anyway (in the food). Vegetables and fruits are carbo*hydrates*. Okay? If you're eating plenty of fruits and vegetables and having a glass or two of water before each meal, that's cool. And if it's hot or if you're thirsty or if you're doing heaps of exercise, take in some more. Water is good. Just don't obsess about it.

By the way, unless you're exercising really hard for up to an hour or more, you don't need all those fancy sports drinks. Plain water is fine. A good rule of thumb is this: if your urine is almost clear, your hydration is okay.

Spreads

Butter or margarine? If it's a very thin scrape, who cares? Actually, I very rarely use either.

On my whole-grain bread, my choices are usually a thin spread of avocado, or some tomato slices, or a touch of olive oil and balsamic vinegar, or a combination of all three. Sometimes I go with hummus.

Why Would You Eat These Foods?

I was going to call this final section of the chapter "Banned Foods," but I don't believe in banning foods, so I've changed the name to "Why Would You Eat These Foods?"

Here, then, are a few foods that you really, truly don't need in the Switch On weeks. Just don't go there.

Croissants

Commercial muesli

Cereals in a box (except for basic oats)

Fruit juice

Soft drinks/soda pop

Muffins

Doughnuts

Reheated foods

Chicken (except skinless breast)

White bread

Cookies/crackers

Fast foods

Butter/margarine

French fries

Other fried foods

Snacks in packets

Dried fruits

Dressings (except a touch of olive oil or oil and vinegar)

Sauces

Lunch meats

Pressed meats

Processed meats

Sausage/salami

Chapter 13

‖‖‖

Put the *F* Back in *Life*

Let's end where we started. In the introduction, I asked you to think about *life*. What a word, isn't it? *L-I-F-E. Life.*

And what a gift. Life is about ego, sure. But life is also about achievement and self-esteem and sunshine. It's about laughter, too—and hugging and negotiating and doings things for other people and enjoying yourself and looking forward to things.

Life is about *please* and *thank you* and doing your best.

Life is all that—and much, much more. So you have to ask yourself: Are you getting the most out of life, or are you cutting corners just to keep up with life's many demands? Have you taken the *F* out of *life*?

By now, having read my earlier discussion, you know what happens when you take the *F* out of *life*. You're left with just a *lie*. Instead of living a lie, like millions of other people around the world, put the *F* back in your life—four *F*s, in fact: family, fun, friendships, faith.

If you had the next three months off—three months free from work, stress, financial concerns, deadlines—which *F*s would you want back in your life to make it a real life and not a lie? I can hear you already: you're muttering a few other *F*-words, aren't you? But here are the four most popular *F*s sampled from thousands of responses I've received from people all over the world.

Family

First among them is family.

My family—my wife, my children, my grandchildren—is my number one priority. I've been married to the same gorgeous girl for more than 40 years, and we have five children and eight wonderful grandchildren. I love my family, and I *need* them. Family members offer great support and unconditional love, which is all we can ask for from life.

Isn't it sad when you consider how many families fall to pieces? I'm sure I don't need to discuss the major reasons for family differences. You know them well. Perhaps you even know them from personal experience. While some family rifts are noisy and tumultuous, neglect can sneak up quietly and be just as destructive. With other things *demanding* our attention, we let family matters slide.

Are *you* so busy with everything else in your life that family has been overshadowed? Where has the balance gone?

Phone your brother or sister—or *any* relative you haven't spoken to in years. Go and have a cup of coffee or a glass of wine together and talk, and then give him or her a huge hug. Rebuild those family bridges.

Family is the first place we all learn to express love, which just happens to be the first step toward experiencing a happy, healthy, wealthy, and wise life.

One of the great fixtures of the longest-living, healthiest people in the world is their lifelong respect for the integrity of the family. When people get old in America, family members often put them in rest homes. What do they do once there? They *rest*. They sit in a La-Z-Boy and watch television all day. Not exactly a great way to spend your Golden Years.

Okinawans, on the other hand, love and support every member of their families—young and old alike. As a matter of fact, there aren't any *old people* in Okinawa. They're known as *elders*—and Okinawans respect and love their elders. There are no rest homes in Okinawa either. The elders stay at home in the village; they remain an integral part of their community, cornerstones of Okinawan families, endless sources of warmth, compassion, and love.

This is just one of the many reasons Okinawans regularly live to their 80s and 90s—and one of the many reasons Okinawans are my heroes. They understand and celebrate and honor the importance of love.

It's impossible to separate love and long life. Having traveled the world, studying and talking with people who enjoy fulfilling and long lives, I know that love is at the center of every good life. You can *love* or *be in love with* someone, or you can *love something* as a momentary experience. Either way, love is related to long life, happiness, and health. Trust me, I'm a doctor. I know what I'm talking about, and science—good old science—backs me up.

One of the scientific explanations for all this lies in the hormone oxytocin. Produced by the hypothalamus (a portion of your brain), oxytocin spikes during moments of intimate connection, including sexual activity. Science can now measure oxytocin levels and tell how in love you are! Increasing oxytocin, which you do by loving abundantly, helps keep your brain young—well, oxytocin along with other hormones and chemicals (such as endorphins, serotonin, and dopamine) and all those micronutrients in plant food.

Talk about good news: lovemaking—that's s-e-x—increases the good hormones in your brain.

We need water. We need food. We need oxygen. We need sex. That's why you're here. Sex is just a fact of life. It's vital—and good for you.

As I noted above, sexual activity increases your oxytocin levels. It also helps you stay in shape, sometimes to the tune of 400 calories per hour. (Two minutes burns only 13 calories, so don't rush things!)

You don't necessarily have to have sex in order to live a long time, but it doesn't hurt. Furthermore, while sex plays a role in helping you achieve a long life, it can also be a barometer of how well you're living. *Loving* well (physically and emotionally) means *living* well.

Let's hope you have a partner, whether it's a companion or a lover or a longtime friend or a family that supports you. If you do have someone who loves you, did you hug him or her—them!—in the last forty-eight hours? Hugging, like sex, can build up the body's feel-good hormones and may reduce the body's bad hormones. When you hug someone you love, that feeling, that warmth, comes out in your relationship.

Remember that old Louis Armstrong song "What a Wonderful World"? It has a verse that goes, "I see friends shaking hands, saying, 'How do you do?' They're really saying, 'I love you.'" What's Louis talking about there? He's talking about social connectedness.

Fun

I ask people all the time, "How are you?" Many of them respond, "Not too bad."

What this tepid response tells me is that they're living only between 30 and 60 percent of their life potential. Everyone's life potential should be closer to the 90 to 100 mark!

I recently ran into an old friend, Bob, in a local shopping center. Bob had trained to be a priest before his life took a different direction. I still sometimes refer to Bob as an apprentice priest. When our paths crossed at the shopping center that day, I asked Bob how he was doing.

"Fabulous!" he replied. "Just great!"

This is how it's supposed to be. Bob adheres to a philosophy that *every* day is a good day. When he wakes up in the morning, he thanks heaven he's alive today.

I wish all those miserable souls out there who moan and groan their way through life would take a lesson from the apprentice priest.

Life is all about attitude, isn't it? It's up to *you* to determine what you want out of life. What are your expectations, and how do you hope to achieve them?

Specifically, what about expectations relating to your health? Are you focused on *life* expectancy or *health* expectancy? As I see it, how long you're going to live isn't what counts. It's how long you expect to be *healthy*. And it's your call. It's under your control.

Remember that the Okinawan Centenarian Study, which I've cited often in this book, showed that genetics accounts for only 30 percent of your health. You control the other 70 percent. Increasing your health expectancy comes down to making health-supportive choices.

In other words, it's not the cards you've been dealt. It's the way you play the game.

What are you afraid of—a little fun and stress-free living?

Have you ever watched the reactions of people at the airport when the airline announces that their flight will be delayed 40 minutes? You'd think their son had crashed the car, their business had gone bust, and World War III had started—all at once. The anguish, the frustration, the abuse.

But who cares, really? What's the point of getting uptight?

Phone through to your destination and tell people what's going on. Go buy a novel or a magazine, and then sit back and relax while workers finish getting the plane ready or the storm passes.

For God's sake, lighten up a little. Try laughing. It's impossible to be angry or annoyed or stressed out when you're laughing.

Like being happy, having fun is a daily decision. So if you're not happy, not having fun, adjust your attitude! As I wrote in chapter 5, "attitude" is the most important word in the English language. It can change your life!

The great thing about a positive attitude is that we positive creatures are definitely in the minority, which means there's a lot more room for us to move and maneuver. On our side, the park is wide open. Imagine if everyone saw the silver lining in the clouds. Imagine if everyone saw the opportunity in adversity. It would be an awful crush.

As it is, though, there's plenty of space to spread your wings. Try it sometime—the freedom feels great. Smile a little and move over to the happy side.

So what about the tough times? Yes, what about them? I'm here to tell you: they have an upside. Very few genuine winners ever come out of *good* times. The successes that emerge from boom times are fleeting—here today, gone tomorrow. It's out of *tough* times that true success emerges. Remember, the pressures on most people are about the same. It's your choice whether you respond positively or negatively.

How do you want to live? Under partly cloudy skies or partly sunny ones? Those expressions mean the same thing, don't they? But why search for the clouds rather than the clear blue sky?

When was the last time you hugged someone? When was the last time you smiled? When was the last time you patted someone on the back for a job well done? When was the last time you did something nice for someone?

How long ago did you and your partner sit and laugh together? At the dinner table? At a movie? The last several movies you went to were probably cops-and-robbers flicks or intense emotional dramas. How about going to a comedy?

Laughter and sex are the two best breakers of stress known to man (and woman). We're not sure whether they're number one and number two, respectively, or number two and number one. But if they come together, that's a sure sign you're getting old!

There are lots of things you can do to find the bright side of life. Laugh. Smile. Share. Love.

Friendships

Let me share an old joke: What's best, a pile of money or a pile of friends? A pile of money: you can always rent a few friends. I love this joke because it underlines the true value of friendship.

As noted above, the Okinawan culture depends on social support systems. Okinawans' entire way of life revolves around their connections with other people.

"But, Doctor," you say. "I have friends, lots of them." This is probably true, but do you have *friendships* with your friends?

When was the last time you actually did something together? When was the last time you gave up some time to talk with a friend, maybe ask for that friend's opinion or advice?

You don't need a lot of friends, but you do need nourishing friends. Don't bother with the toxic kind. One of the worst things in your life is the toxicity that builds when you're around negative people. Again, which do you want to focus on?

Faith

Essential to a fulfilling life is a connection with a higher being, an inherent belief that there is goodness in the world. Being spiritual is a part of human life, and a part of love.

"Well, that sounds great, Doctor, but what the heck is spirituality?" Simply put, spirituality is a belief in something bigger than yourself. And it's a reason to exist.

I'm not talking about religion here. I'm talking about something far less structured—something that is an inherent part of the lives of the longest-living and healthiest people on earth.

We need to learn from them. They share their lives with one another, supporting friends and family alike, with an inherent belief that in all human beings there is some goodness. Each individual's measure of goodness comes from how he or she relates to and takes care of other people.

Compare this to how we measure success in Western cultures. A lot of businesspeople in the world today think only about wins and losses—as in "I win; you lose." That's how business folks make money. Unfortunately, success in the Western world is all about money and other numbers. They're just part of the deal. How much? How many? How big?

Spirituality, on the other hand, is not just part of the deal; it's the biggest part of the deal. It's not win-lose, but win-win.

Spiritual people are happy and contented people. They're kind and often think of others. They're very good at giving.

These initial four *F*s are terribly important. Think about the power of family, fun, friendships, and faith as you Love, Laugh, and Eat your way to 100.

But also think about another four *F*s, which I include here based on what we've learned about the longest-living, healthiest cultures. These new four *F*s help round out a good life: fiber, fish, fruit, (and vegetables), fitness. If they sound familiar, it's because they overlap nicely with the elements of the ACE protocol.

Just as these four *F*s work in collaboration, the magic of the ACE protocol lies in the combination of all three of its elements: Activity, Coping, Eating. They're all tied together. You need to involve your body, your mind, and your mouth to be successful.

Life should be a total body experience. It's your mind. It's your physical form. It's your spirit. It's also your work life and your family life. It's your leisure. It's your community.

The road to a happy, healthy, wealthy, and wise life begins with *you*.

When it comes to Loving, Laughing, and Eating your way to 100, the choice is entirely up to you. What kind of life do you want to live? How long do you want to be healthy?

Acknowledgments

Inspiration is what I have needed to put something into words that can help people live a better life. I have been inspired by several people and a sincere thank-you is due to them on a continuing basis. A division is possible: heroes and OGTs (other genuine thank-yous).

My three heroes—

—my wife and best friend, Sue, the most amazing person on the planet.

—Jack Nicklaus, who proved that aging and maturing does not prevent you being a champion, performing under pressure on both the sporting field and in life.

—George Burns, who showed me that loving and laughing your way to 100 is a great way to go.

A special thank-you to—

—the longest-living, healthiest people on earth, the Okinawans.

—the many people who have successfully followed their and my principles to feel and look younger, for longer in life.

—our five, fabulous children (and their children) who can share laughter, and clothing, with their mother!

—the wonderful people at PBS, especially Bob Marty, the creative, lateral thinker, and his brother Bill.

—Miles Doyle, who made the physical creation of this book possible. And all the other great people at HarperOne, including Gideon Weil, Suzanne Quist, Melinda Mullin, Amy VanLangen, Claudia Boutote, and Mark Tauber.

I am indebted, and trust we can assist you to raise the bar, to Love, Laugh, and Eat your way to 100!

|||||||||||||||||||||||||||||||||||||||||||||||||||||||||||||||||||||||||||||||||||||||||||||||||||||

Maybe You Need an Oil Change?

*O*il in cooking is very important. Think of oil as a lubricant and in particular cases, a flavor enhancer.

Used sparingly, oils are even healthy!

Most people consider *fat* as the enemy, but a quick trip around the world's various populations shows that saturated fats aren't so good, polyunsaturated fats are reasonable, monounsaturated fats are good, and trans fats are a total disaster!

Animal fats are saturated fats, so less is better. Some plant fats/oils are mainly saturated—coconut oil, palm oil, and cocoa butter—although of the trio, cocoa and chocolate (especially dark chocolate) are okay in small amounts. I said small amounts.

Animal fats are usually solid at room temperature so a good rule of thumb is this—the harder the fat on your plate, the harder it is in your arteries!

Most plant food oils and fish oils are polyunsaturated fats, which are liquid at room temperature. They don't stick—they move through your arteries and tissues.

There are omega-3 and omega-6 oils, and our levels have gotten way out of balance in recent times. We need more 3s and less 6s. So more fish oil and more olive oils. Flaxseed oil is good too.

The best examples of foods containing a decent whack of mono-unsaturated fats—often referred to as Mediterranean fats—are olives, olive oils, avocado, almond oil, and canola oil.

Popeye was on the ball with good friend Olive Oyl and his spinach intake was also to be applauded.

Here's a table noting various oils in decreasing order of mono-unsaturated (good) fat content.

Type of Oil/Fat	Percent Fat (approx.)		
	Saturated	Poly-unsaturated	Mono-unsaturated
Olive oil	14	12	74
Almond oil	8	19	73
Canola oil	7	35	58
Peanut oil	18	33	47
Rice bran oil	20	33	47
Margarine tub	17	37	46
Sesame oil	15	43	42
Palm oil	52	10	38
Cocoa butter	63	3	34
Butter	66	4	30
Wheat germ oil	20	50	30
Butter, whipped	69	3	28
Corn oil	13	62	25
Soybean oil	15	61	24
Sunflower oil	11	69	20
Walnut oil	14	67	19
Flaxseed oil	9	72	19
Safflower oil	9	78	13
Coconut oil	92	2	6

As long as you're using fats and oils sparingly, it would be fine to use any of the following good oils. These oils are low in saturated fats and trans fats. Some have a high concentration of mono-unsaturated fats such as olive oil. Choose corn oil, safflower oil, sunflower oil, soy oil, or canola oil if you wish to fry foods, because these oils have a higher smoke point. It is best not to fry with olive oil. Its smoke point is only about 375 degrees.

Good Cooking Oils	Bad Cooking Oils
Olive oil	Vegetable shortening
Canola oil	Hard margarine
Safflower oil	Butter
Nonhydrogenated soft margarine	Palm oil
	Palm kernel oil
Corn oil	Coconut oil
Peanut oil	

Remember that all oils have about 120 calories per tablespoon. (You could eat two small apples for that number of calories.) The first rule with cooking oils is to use as little as possible. Oil is fat, and too much fat can contribute to obesity.

Use a nonstick pan to fry meat and add one tablespoon of oil for the equivalent of a four-person meal. If you have heart disease or are at high risk for heart disease, olive oil and canola oil are smart choices.

If you're looking for a burst of flavor, choose a stronger oil, such as sesame, peanut, or walnut. Use these oils in salad dressings instead of cooking, because they burn easily. Peanut and walnut oil also give a mild, nutty flavor to salad dressings when mixed with balsamic or other flavored vinegar.

Corn, safflower, and sunflower oils are high in polyunsaturated fats, but should still be used sparingly.

Boost your omega-3 fatty acid intake by choosing walnut oil or flaxseed oil. Omega-3 fatty acids are also found in fatty fish, such as salmon, trout, and mackerel, and are important for maintaining a healthy heart and blood vessel system. You can't really use flaxseed oil for cooking.

If you're looking for a cooking oil to fry foods, choose one that won't burn quickly. Corn, safflower, and soya oils are excellent choices. Remember that fried foods absorb quite a bit of the oil they are cooked in and therefore are much higher in calories and fat.

Now let's take a closer look at olive oil.

Good olive oil is highly prized—not only for its health benefits, but also for its wonderful flavor. The best oil is a blend of oil from a mixture of red-ripe (not green and not fully ripe) olives and a smaller proportion of oil from green olives of a different variety. Cold-pressing, a chemical-free process using only pressure, produces a higher quality of olive oil, which is naturally lower in acidity. If you are a serious student of olive oil, it's important to check labels for the percentage of acidity, grade of oil, and country of origin. The level of acidity is a key factor in choosing fine olive oil, along with color, flavor, and aroma.

Extra-Virgin Olive Oil

Cold-pressed, the result of the first pressing of the olives with only 1 percent acid. Extra-virgin olive oil is considered the finest and fruitiest—and the most expensive. It ranges from a crystalline champagne color to greenish golden to bright green. Generally the deeper the color, the more intense the olive flavor.

Virgin Olive Oil

Also a first-pressed oil with a slightly higher acidity level of between 1 and 3 percent.

Fino Olive Oil

Fino olive oil is a blend of extra-virgin olive oil and virgin olive oils. "Fino" is Italian for "fine."

Light Olive Oil

This contains the same amount of beneficial monounsaturated fats as regular olive oil, but due to the refining process, it is lighter in color and has essentially no flavor. This makes it a good choice for baking and other purposes where its heavy flavor might not be desirable. Light olive oil also has a higher smoking point, making it a prime candidate for high-heat cooking.

Olive Oil Storage

Store olive oil in a cool, dark place for up to six months, or in the refrigerator for up to a year. Check the label for bottling. Olive oil does not improve with age like fine wine and is best when used during the first six months after pressing. Refrigerated or very cold olive oil will become cloudy, but will become clear again when brought to room temperature. Be sure it's kept in an airtight container or bottle. Use higher quality forms of olive oil for flavor and lower grades for high-heat applications.

Olive Oil Health Benefits

Olive oil is a staple of the traditional Mediterranean diet. Although as much as 40 percent of total daily calories are from fat, cardiovascular diseases are not generally found in mature Italians unless they have been influenced by the Western style of eating. Olive oil is also a good source of antioxidants. Eating fish a few times a week similarly increases levels of omega-3 fatty acids. Eating red meat sparingly is also a positive. The fats found in olive oil are digested and metabolized more efficiently than other fats.

Olives have been used in Mediterranean appetizers for thousands of years. Green olives are often stuffed, while black olives may be soaked in oil. Olives of different color varieties are used in numerous Mediterranean dishes to add a distinct flavor.

Just another lesson we can learn from our neighbors in a multicultural environment.

Index

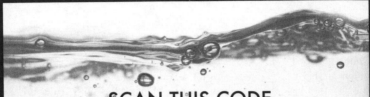

SCAN THIS CODE
WITH YOUR SMARTPHONE TO BE LINKED TO
THE BONUS MATERIALS FOR

LOVE, LAUGH, AND EAT

on the Elixir website,
where you can also find information about other
healthy living books and related materials.

YOU CAN ALSO TEXT
LOVELAUGH to READIT (732348)

to be sent a link to the Elixir website.

 Facebook.com/elixirliving   Twitter.com/elixirliving   www.elixirliving.com